Praise for *Helpir*

"*Helping Baby Sleep* has two essential ingredients: practical advice about infant sleep garnered from neurobiological, social-emotional, and attachment literatures, and a compassionate, sensitive attitude toward both infants and parents. Translating diverse scientific findings into applicable tools, Gethin and Macgregor encourage positive and gentle practices that enhance the quality of infant sleep and strengthen the parent-infant relationship. A must-read that sheds light on one of the most common parenting issues of infancy and early childhood."

> —Hiram E. Fitzgerald, PhD, former executive director of the
> World Association for Infant Mental Health (1992–2008) and
> co-editor of the *WAIMII Handbook of Infant Mental Health*

"Gethin and Macgregor have boldly and successfully waded into the complex issues of infant sleep, creating a guide that gives hope and support to parents. Grounded in common sense and respect for the infant, the lessons in this book are both comforting and empowering, showing parents how they can gently guide the emotional experiences of their babies. How remarkable that a book could have these features and still represent cutting-edge research. A magnificent gift to mothers and fathers—superb."

> —Michael Trout, MA, director of the Infant-Parent Institute

"This is a beautiful book, rich with empathy for babies and parents, and also practical and down-to-earth. Infants are not our enemies. They are not feral creatures to be tamed, domesticated, and programmed to become adults who are obedient and placatory. When we respect their individuality and respond to what they are trying to tell us, we help them develop social skills, grow in self-confidence, and give and receive love."

> —Sheila Kitzinger, author of *Understanding Your Crying Baby*

"What makes *Helping Baby Sleep* beautiful is that it does not focus on manipulating infant behavior, but on the more important issue of creating a secure and sensitive relationship between parent and child. The authors present helping your baby learn to sleep as part of a larger philosophy and approach to parenting—one that is grounded in responsive emotional support. Gethin and Macgregor explain how parents can provide their babies with feelings of safety and comfort, which helps them (and the rest of the family) fall asleep."

—Bert Powell, Glen Cooper, and Kent Hoffman, co-founders of the Circle of Security®: Early Intervention Program for Parents and Children

"Gethin and Macgregor's work is an outstanding example of translating very recent advances in the developmental sciences into sensitive, empathic models of child rearing. Their carefully researched and clearly explained approach to the important matter of infant sleep behaviors is based on a deep understanding of current research, which demonstrates that attachment interactions directly impact the development of the infant brain. I highly recommend this important book."

—Allan N. Schore, PhD, author of *Affect Dysregulation and Disorders of the Self* and *Affect Regulation and the Repair of the Self*

"In *Helping Baby Sleep*, Gethin and Macgregor address all the major issues we parents fret about: Is co-sleeping okay? Can I put my baby in a crib and not scar her for life? Why doesn't he sleep through the night? How can I get her to stop crying? Am I doing anything wrong? Will my baby survive my parenting? Using a warm, conversational style, they soothe away our worries with practical, gentle, and easy-to-follow advice. This book should be given to mothers and fathers at every baby shower."

—Meredith F. Small, PhD, author of *Our Babies, Ourselves: How Biology and Culture Shape the Way We Parent*

"I can't imagine any parent reading this informed, wise, and power-fully argued book, and ever wanting to use controlled crying again."

—Steve Biddulph, author of *The Secret of Happy Children* and *Raising Boys*

"Much advice about infant sleep is both unrealistic and harshly neglect-ful of babies' needs. [*Helping Baby Sleep*] is very different: Anni and Beth have a wonderful, warm way of combining scientific evidence against harsh practices such as controlled crying, with the wisdom gleaned from their own mothering experiences. They unapologetically advo-cate for the baby's well-being while also acknowledging parents' very real needs for support. If [*Helping Baby Sleep*] was mandatory reading for anyone caring for babies . . . . [children] would be free to reach their potential for emotional and intellectual well-being."

—Pinky McKay, author of *Sleeping Like a Baby*

"This is an important book for parents because it puts babies' sleep in the context of research about infant development. There are many books that give suggestions about how to 'train babies to sleep' but none that I know of that give parents the information to make their decisions about sleep, taking into account their babies' developmental needs."

—Pam Linke, author and national president of the Australian Association for Infant Mental Health

"At last—an antidote to the current vogue for leaving babies to cry! Many parents have felt intuitively that this cannot be the way to deal with their infants, but too often they are encouraged to ignore their feelings and to ignore baby's distress signals as well."

—Carolyn Quadrio, MBBS, PhD, professor of psychiatry at the University of New South Wales

Helping
Baby Sleep

Helping Baby Sleep

The Science and Practice of Gentle Bedtime Parenting

Anni Gethin, PhD, and Beth Macgregor

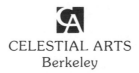

CELESTIAL ARTS
Berkeley

Published in the United States by Celestial Arts, an imprint of the
Crown Publishing Group, a division of Random House, Inc., New York.
www.crownpublishing.com
www.tenspeed.com

Celestial Arts and the Celestial Arts colophon are registered trademarks
of Random House, Inc.

First published as *Helping Your Baby to Sleep* in Australia in 2007
by Finch Publishing Pty. Ltd.

Interior photographs courtesy of Finch Publishing, the authors, and the
Australian Breastfeeding Association

Library of Congress Cataloging-in-Publication Data
Gethin, Anni.
 Helping baby sleep : the science and practice of gentle bedtime parenting /
Anni Gethin and Beth Macgregor.
    p. cm.
 Includes bibliographical references and index.
 Summary: "A baby sleep book that advocates responsive parenting and cites
research in infant neural and emotional development"—Provided by publisher.
 1. Infants—Sleep. 2. Infants—Development. 3. Parent and infant 4. Child rearing.
I. Macgregor, Beth. II. Title.

RJ506.S55G48 2009
649'.122—dc22

                                                2009010739
ISBN 978-1-58761-340-1 (pbk.)

Printed in the United States of America
Cover and text design by Chloe Rawlins
10 9 8 7 6 5 4 3 2 1
First North American Edition, 2009

For our parents

Contents

Acknowledgments

This book has been made possible by the contributions of people who feel as deeply about babies' sleep-time needs as we do. Their generosity will help parents feel confident to nurture their babies and feel reassured that they are not alone.

We would like to begin by thanking Sue Cox for encouraging us to write this book. We also want to thank the many parents who kindly shared their stories and wisdom with us. Many of these parents allowed us to include photos of their precious children, as did other generous souls. We are also grateful to the Australian Breastfeeding Association for sharing so many lovely photos. We extend thanks to Michelle Barnes, Caroline Kochenborger, Erika Nentwich, and Cindy Wright, with a special thank-you to Yvette O'Dowd.

We are indebted to the many experts who so generously corresponded with us and agreed to be quoted. Their perspectives will give parents valuable insights into their children's development and emotional needs. Thanks go to Dr. Harry Edhouse, Dr. Vicky Flory, Dr. Karin Grossmann, Joan Hailes, Dr. Daniel Hughes, Anne Kohn, Dr. Isla Lonie, Pinky McKay, Marianne Nicholson, Dr. Carolyn Quadrio, and Dr. Allan N. Schore.

We are grateful for the conversations we had with other specialists who supported us and shared their wisdom with us: Leanne Clarke, Dr. Robyn Dolby, Barb Glare, Dr. Karleen Gribble, Robin Grille, Margaret Hope, Lisa Liber, Pam Linke, Dr. Carol Newnham, Elizabeth Pantley, and Macall Gordon.

Some of these people also gave us valuable comments on early drafts of the manuscript. We extend a special thanks to Lauren Porter and to our other readers, Jo Butler and Kate Dent Rennie, who provided important feedback on the manuscript.

We are thankful for the work of our Australian publisher, Rex Finch, and editor, Kathryn Lamberton, in helping us to craft a book that will be accessible to parents and of interest to professionals. We are grateful for the invaluable support we have received from our editors at Celestial Arts—Clancy Drake, Genoveva Llosa, and Ashley Thompson—in preparing this book for publication in North America.

Other supporters have been our dear friends who have shared many cups of tea, glasses of wine, and long, inspiring conversations. Thanks to Danielle Conroy, Jeanette Crawford, Jane Elix, Julie Grove, Meredith Hope, Amanda Hunt, and Paula Keating.

We would also like to thank Beth's husband, Mark; the father of Anni's children, Alex; and Luke and Matthew's grandparents, Ronda, Carmen, and Ian. They cared for our beloved children while we hid in libraries and cafés with our laptops—without their help this book would not have been written. We are also grateful to our children, Zac, Ben, Karl, and Luke and Matthew, who were largely patient with us as we focused on creating this book. They have opened our hearts to a love that is deeper and truer than we have ever known.

Foreword

New parents are often surprised to learn that babies don't always sleep like we do—in one long slice, once a night, and at a convenient and regular time. It's a *good* thing they don't—it's too long for them to go without nourishment, and they are programmed to rouse from time to time to seek out cuddles and reassurance that adults are close by.

Every parent should understand and accept this. Then, when our babies need us to lie down with them to fall asleep, or when they wake several times a night (as most do), we will realize this is quite normal and healthy. And we will begin to adjust our lives to take it into account. In time, gradually and with support and care, parents and babies find a rhythm that works for them both.

The problem with controlled crying is the mind-set that it arises from: that babies need us to *control* them; that since we already put insane demands on adults in our society, it should also be possible to do so with infants; and if it doesn't work, to find a quick fix.

In the sixty years that controlled crying has been in and out of fashion, it's my belief, and the belief of many psychiatrists and child developmentalists, that it has done great harm to the mental health of babies and to the trusting connection parents want to create with their children.*

The agencies that support and teach controlled crying have the best of motives and care deeply about the distressed and exhausted

---

* Australian Association for Infant Mental Health, *Position Paper 1: Controlled Crying* (Revised March 2004), www.aaimhi.org/documents/position%20 papers/controlled_crying.pdf (accessed December 2008).

parents who come to them for help. But in advocating such techniques, they opt for a method that impacts the baby rather than one that works with parents to help meet their own and their babies' needs in better ways. Cortisol testing from saliva has verified what common sense and kindness also tell us—that infants feel acute stress when they are left to cry alone for more than a moment or two. And stress harms them. Parents suffering from sleep deprivation need practical support and investments of more time and human energy. And they need help to understand their babies.

Fortunately, this excellent book, and the resources it directs parents to, offers ways of working with babies' sleep patterns and of creating the conditions for better sleep, without endangering infants' mental health or damaging their experience of being loved and safe.

Anni Gethin and Beth Macgregor are experienced mothers and researchers, and Beth is also a highly skilled helper who worked with parents in crisis for many years. They present fascinating research into how babies develop and how infant sleep works. They give plenty of examples and anecdotes culled from parents. And best of all, their methods are adaptable and loving, even if they mean spending more time, more care, and more energy on parents and their babies. They treat parents and babies as precious, and I thank them for doing so.

—*Steve Biddulph*

Introduction:
Hear the Babies Crying

But what am I?
An infant crying in the night:
An infant crying for the light:
And with no language but a cry.[1]
ALFRED, LORD TENNYSON

This book is about responsive parenting. It is about how babies thrive when parents are sensitive to their needs—during the day and the night. It looks at baby sleep and shows that babies wake up at night and need help to settle for many good reasons, as frustrating as this may be to their parents.

Sleep training, which aims to teach children to fall asleep independently by leaving them to cry without comfort, is the opposite of our approach. It is hugely popular among parents and widely recommended by health professionals. Sleep training takes many forms and is known by different names, including *cry it out, Ferberizing, progressive waiting, crying down, the extinction method, graduated extinction, partial ignoring, cold turkey, controlled comforting,* and *controlled crying.* However, an explosion of new research in early childhood development in recent years has led many to ask: is sleep training really something we should be doing to our children?

This book is in two parts. In part 1: "Science—Research Supports Responsive Parenting," we examine baby sleep, showing why babies wake at night and why they need help to settle. This is followed by a discussion of love and bonding—how responsive parenting sets up babies for life (and makes them less likely to cause trouble when they are teenagers!). Then we journey into the baby brain and find out how the neurological structures that let us feel emotions and cope with stress are built in the first years of life. Next we have a good look at sleep training—what it is and why it is so distressing for babies and their parents.

In part 2: "Practice—Gentle Ways to Help Your Baby (and You)," we offer guidance on how to gently settle your baby, providing effective techniques and routines for children of different ages. This is followed by an exploration of common sleep problems and corresponding coping methods that will help you and your baby sleep better. We then outline the six essential elements of responsive parenting—in which children's needs and feelings are taken seriously and attended to. Responding to another's needs is much easier when we feel taken care of, so we conclude this part by discussing how parents can receive the nurturing and support they require.

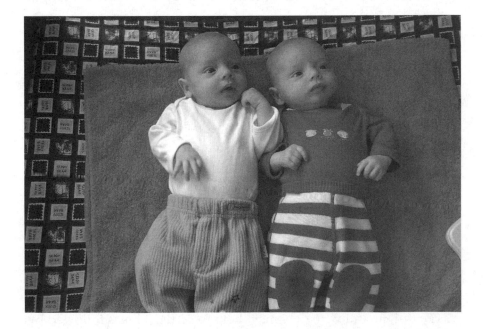

How We Became Concerned

We first became concerned about sleep training in the early nineties when we were at university. Beth was studying psychology; Anni was studying education and adjusting to being a first-time mom to baby Zac. At this stage, all we knew was that sleep training *felt* wrong—why on earth would a parent be told not to pick up a crying baby? We were curious to find out what child development research said about leaving children to cry for extended periods of time. What we found alarmed us. There was mounting evidence that failing to respond to a crying child can cause stress and harm to that child, yet there was no credible research into the impact of sleep training on children's emotional well-being or brain development. No one could confidently say "Sleep training does not harm babies."

After completing her degree, Beth spent five years working with abused and neglected children and their parents, and she went on to train professionals who work with parents and children. She learned how deeply babies and children need their parents to show them empathy and how this is more likely to happen when parents have a lot of good support. She had two children, Luke and Matthew, delightful boys who were still waking at night long after most baby books said they should be sleeping through. Anni had two more children, Ben and Karl, and embarked on a PhD in population health, examining social and economic influences on health. Her second baby, Ben, was very sensitive and was a terrible sleeper who truly tested the parenting skills of Anni and her partner. It was particularly heartbreaking for Anni to hear stories of people using sleep training on high-need babies like Ben—it seemed to her that these babies would suffer terribly.

Is Sleep Training Risky?

Over the years, as we have read more and new research has become available, our concern about sleep training has increased. This research clearly shows that sleep training has to be risky for children: being separated from their parents and having no one respond to their cries can be deeply stressful and even traumatic.[2] We found that babies whose cries are ignored can learn to look strong and independent, but inside they can feel insecure and anxious that their moms and dads will not be there for them when needed. These anxieties can last a lifetime. We learned that babies and small children see themselves as the cause of their experiences, so they can come to believe that *they* are to blame when no one comes to comfort them. We discovered that being left to cry without comfort can put a lot of stress on babies' developing brains, possibly permanently affecting the way they respond to stress in later life.

When we published articles and spoke at conferences about our concerns, and talked to more and more people about what children actually experienced during sleep training, we became even more troubled. *Sleep training* is a benign term that describes a deeply painful—even brutal—experience for babies and young children. The following are just some of the things we heard:

> My daughter stood in her crib crying and shrieking and shaking violently all over, screaming for me and even trying to climb out of the crib. . . . She was absolutely terrified because she was alone and didn't know where we were.

> My baby works himself into such a state I'm afraid he's going to stop breathing.[3]

> When I let him cry, he got hysterical and I ended up crying myself. It was just not right, and it didn't work like magic either.

> We had one night we called the "prisoner of war night" because our son was sitting in his crib hanging on to the bars wailing

and falling asleep between wails with his head drooped. He did it for nearly an hour. It's so hard not to go comfort them. We kept at it and he eventually gave up and went to sleep.

I worry as she just stands in her cot [crib] screaming and screaming. . . . The crying isn't so bad, it's the screaming.

[Nine days of sleep training] doesn't seem to be working. . . . My son is on his third nap of the day. He has screamed through all of them.

The longest Alexander has ever cried was two and a half hours, and the only reason he stopped is that I got him up. He could have and would have screamed longer. The kid has more will than we do; that's why [sleep training] didn't work for us. He also vomited and there isn't really anything you can do besides listen or check for it or decide to leave them in it.

As these stories show, babies are experiencing immense anguish and suffering in the name of sleep. One of the world's leading researchers into children's emotional development, associate professor Edward Z. Tronick has shown how dramatically babies are affected when their parents refuse to respond to them. Yet he says, "People don't want to believe that a child could be so hurt—or that we could be so hurtful."[4] Even babies for whom the sleep training process seems relatively rapid nearly always cry and become distressed, usually for several nights. It is uncommon for sleep training to change children's sleep habits permanently, so it is often repeated several times. Few parents are not deeply upset by the process of sleep training their baby.

Why Do Parents Use Sleep Training?

Despite almost universal distress when implementing sleep training, the techniques remain very popular. This is not surprising given that parents receive advice to sleep train from trusted professionals, and they are promised that it cannot harm their babies. There are many seemingly good reasons why parents choose to use it; for example, their baby does not get enough sleep or wakes up five times a night in search of a pacifier. Other parents are exhausted from broken sleep and use sleep training to relieve the stress of chronic tiredness.

In other cases, parents are fearful that if they continue to respond to their baby at bedtime, he will never learn to sleep through the night or go to sleep by himself. This view is often presented to parents by health professionals. In these cases, sleep training is used to prevent children from learning to rely on their parents at sleep time and during the night, because these behaviors are (falsely) seen to be problematic.

Our view is that sleep training is akin to the advice that used to be given to parents to breast-feed their babies every four hours and not a minute sooner. Conscientious parents followed this advice, despite many babies screaming in hunger, pain, and distress. Science has now shown how rigid feeding schedules do not meet babies' biological need to feed frequently. It is our hope that professionals and parents will become aware of *why* babies sleep differently than adults, rely on their parents at bedtime, and require comfort when they are distressed. Once infants' biological needs and makeup are better understood, information about gentle ways to modify babies' sleep will become more readily available, and parents will be freed to respond to their crying babies.

Why Do We Need to Understand Normal Baby Sleep Needs?

In many instances, sleep training is about fixing parents' problems—not genuine baby sleep problems. Some popular parenting guides refer to normal sleep behavior, such as night waking and needing help to settle to sleep, as the child having a "problem" or "disorder" that needs "treatment."[5] While we might prefer that our babies be independent at night, dependency on parents during their first years is part of babies' biological design. It is normal for babies and toddlers to need us as much as they do, to wake during the night and need reassurance that their beloved parents are still nearby. It is also normal for all babies and toddlers to have periods when they are more wakeful, such as when they are undergoing developmental changes, learning to crawl or walk, teething, having visitors, or traveling. Babies also vary in the amount of sleep they need—which means that some babies are happy to have *less* than the books say they should.

While it's true that sleep is important and that some babies genuinely have trouble getting enough sleep, allowing babies to cry should not be the preferred way to solve sleep problems. Babies' inability to sleep can sometimes be due to hidden physical problems, such as ear infections, food sensitivities, or the effects of a difficult birth. Parents need support to examine each of these issues carefully. As one mother testifies:

> The nurse, pediatrician, and sleep clinic all told me my twelve-month-old daughter just needed to learn how to sleep and that it was my fault for feeding her at night. . . . None of them ever suggested that there might actually be a reason for her being a poor sleeper or really talked to me about it—this controlled crying was just the answer to everything. . . . We tried it for two weeks, and she screamed for two hours every time she was put to bed, and after two weeks we gave up and went to a family bed. She was diagnosed with chronic glue ear [middle ear infection] at twenty-two months and she had had no other symptoms—a big part of the cause of her sleep problems. I really, really regret controlled crying.

Some children simply have high needs, such as Anni's son Ben, because they are born with nervous systems that make them super-sensitive to their environment. These babies need intensive, sensitive, and patient care. Other babies who have trouble sleeping may need gentle sleep techniques such as those discussed in chapters 5 and 6.

Does Sleep Training Meet Children's Emotional Needs?

Although sleep training does work to change some children's sleep behavior in the short term,[6] bringing about change by causing a child to be distressed can never be considered a success. Contrary to what many professionals tell parents, babies don't cry during sleep training simply because they are tired—they cry because they experience intense emotional pain. Parents should be encouraged to avoid causing their babies emotional pain just as diligently as they avoid inflicting physical pain. Something—well, someone—has been lost in this effort to mold babies' sleep habits. In all of this talk about sleeplessness, sleep loss, and sleep problems, we've lost sight of the babies, of their need—and right—to feel loved and cherished and safe. Of course children need sleep. They also need to feel secure; they have the right to have their physical *and* emotional needs taken seriously. Refusing comfort to distressed babies is akin to refusing them food when they are hungry. It can never be justified.

So, when facing issues with their children's sleep, parents are encouraged to ask the wrong question. It shouldn't be "How can I change my child's sleep habits?"; it should be "Is it possible to change my child's sleep habits while still helping her feel loved and lovable?" Only if the answer to this question is *yes* should the *how* be asked. It is in this spirit that we offer alternative sleep ideas and resources for parents.

This book brings together research in early childhood development, normal baby sleep, baby emotions, and baby neurology, and is illustrated by the experiences of many parents who have struggled through sleepless nights. Parents have generously shared their stories with us through surveys and personal communication. We also quote parents from Internet forums across the world. The names of some parents and children have been changed to protect their privacy.

In this book, we use both male and female pronouns to refer to babies; we alternate *he* and *she* throughout each chapter. We know that families come in many different forms, and while most babies live with their moms and dads, many don't: one parent, stepparents, foster parents, same-sex parents, or grandparents may take care of them, for example. For the sake of simplicity, though, we generally refer to parents as "mom and dad."

NOTES

1. Alfred, Lord Tennyson, "LIV," *In Memoriam*, ed. Erik Gray (New York: W. W. Norton & Company, 2004), 39–40.

2. Jude Cassidy and Phillip R. Shaver, eds., *Handbook of Attachment: Theory, Research, and Clinical Applications* (New York: Guilford Press, 1999); and Allan N. Schore, *Affect Regulation and the Origin of the Self: The Neurobiology of Emotional Development* (Hillsdale, New Jersey: Lawrence Erlbaum Associates, 1994).

3. Marce Viotto, *It's Time to Sleep: How to Get Your Child Sleeping Like a Baby* (Melbourne, Australia: Hybrid, 2004), 36.

4. Edward Z. Tronick, quoted in Deborah Blum, *Love at Goon Park: Harry Harlow and the Science of Affection* (New York: Berkley Publishing Group, 2002), 262.

5. Richard Ferber, *Solve Your Child's Sleep Problems* (St. Leonards, Australia: Dorling Kindersley, 1999), 18; and Brian Symon, *Silent Nights: Overcoming Sleep Problems in Babies and Children* (South Melbourne, Australia: Oxford University Press, 1998), 67.

6. Harriet Hiscock and Melissa Wake, "Randomised Controlled Trial of Behavioural Infant Sleep Intervention to Improve Infant Sleep and Maternal Mood," *British Medical Journal* 324 (May 2002): 1062–1065.

PART 1: SCIENCE

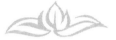

Research Supports Responsive Parenting

CHAPTER 1

Why Babies Wake through the Night

Golden slumber kiss your eyes,
Smiles await you when you rise.
Sleep, pretty baby, do not cry,
And I'll sing you a lullaby.

Care you know not,
Therefore sleep,
While I o'er you watch do keep.
Sleep, pretty darling, do not cry,
And I will sing a lullaby.
TRADITIONAL LULLABY, BASED
ON A POEM BY THOMAS DEKKER[1]

Tired! So very tired. One of the many lessons babies teach their parents is the true meaning of being tired. Dancing all night, cramming for exams, working late evenings—nothing comes close to the sustained sleep disruption potential of a little baby human. In fact, parental tiredness is the main reason so many parents seek advice about how to help their babies sleep through the night—they would do almost anything for a night of uninterrupted sleep!

For better or worse, the baby sleep-wake story is not nearly as simple as that. Everybody wakes up during the night, but older children and adults usually go back to sleep, often not noticing that they've woken up at all. Babies, too, wake up at night, but they need their parents' help to get back to sleep for many reasons.

Parents receive all sorts of misinformation about baby sleep. They might be told that a baby should sleep through the night at six weeks, or maybe three months, or six months. Some people even claim that when a baby reaches a particular weight, there is no reason for her to wake up at night. Many people are not sure what *sleeping through* actually means—is it the five hours defined by some health professionals or eight hours like adults? In fact, there are so many stories about baby sleep that today's parents can get very confused about what is normal and what is not. This confusion means that parents can be more easily persuaded to let their babies cry themselves to sleep; after all, they've been told authoritatively that their baby is now ready to sleep through the night.

Unfortunately, just because advice comes from a health professional doesn't mean it is necessarily accurate or helpful. The developmental psychologists and authors of *How Babies Think: The Science of Childhood* observe the following:

> Assorted quacks, con artists, and bullies have been happy to give advice, often invoking scientific authority. There is a largely dishonorable history of "expert" advice to mothers. To

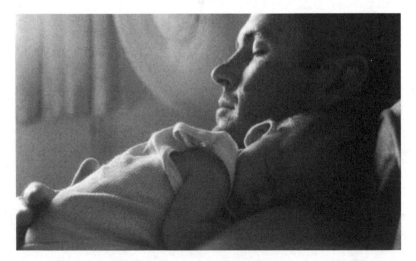

a developmental scientist, the most striking thing about most of this advice is how removed it was from any real empirical evidence or experimental research.[2]

In this chapter, we look at what normal baby sleep really is, why most babies find it difficult to settle themselves to sleep, and why they wake up at night. We also look at how harshly interfering with the normal maturing of sleep biology may carry long-term risks.

You can be reassured that all children will eventually learn how to sleep through the night—but there is no magic age or magic weight at which this should happen. Also, like adults, babies vary in the amount of sleep they need. You may find that you need to ride out the sleep-interrupted nights for a while longer, or you may find that something will help your baby sleep more soundly, as we shall see in later chapters.

What Is Normal Baby Sleep?

When researching this book, we examined the scientific literature about baby sleep and night waking to find out what babies really do when it comes to sleep. We were quite surprised at how different the research findings are compared to information often given to parents. For example, you may have been told that your baby's health will be compromised if he doesn't sleep a certain number of hours during the day and night. Such claims are based on estimates and averages. Research shows that for a given age, individual babies' sleep needs vary quite widely—with differences in total sleep being as much as eight hours; for instance, one baby sleeps ten hours a day, while another sleeps eighteen (see "Sleep Hours by Age" table on page 16). Also, these differences in hours of sleep seem to be largely a matter of individual need and have been shown to have no impact on developmental outcomes such as growth.[3] While helping your baby have all the sleep he needs is important, trying to make him sleep more than he needs can create unnecessary bedtime battles—or even sleep problems.

Sleep Hours by Age: 24-Hour Period (Including Naps)

Age	Average Hours of Sleep	50% of Babies	Range of Nearly All Babies
1 month	14–15	13–16	9–19
3 months	14–15	13–16	10–19
6 months	14	13–15.5	10.5–18
9 months	14	13–15	10.5–17.5
12 months	14	13–15	11.5–16.5
18 months	13.5	13–14.5	11–16
24 months	13	12.5–14	11–15.5

Sources: Ivo Iglowstein, Oskar G. Jenni, Luciano Molinari, and Remo H. Largo, "Sleep Duration from Infancy to Adolescence: Reference Values and Generational Trends," *Pediatrics* 111, no. 2 (February 2003): 302–307; and summarized data from www.parentingscience.com/baby-sleep-requirements.html (accessed August 31, 2008).

Other research shows just how common it is for babies and toddlers to wake during the night and need help getting back to sleep:[4]

- At three months of age, around 80 percent of babies wake up at night and need their parents' help to get back to sleep.

- At six months, about 75 percent of babies regularly wake up at night and need help to go back to sleep.

- Around one year of age, approximately 50 percent of babies sometimes wake up at night and need help to return to sleep.

- Up to four years old, about a third of children will sometimes wake up at night and need help to go back to sleep.

- Many babies who are sleeping through the night will start waking and crying for a parent again, particularly around nine months of age (when separation anxiety begins to develop).

- Some babies whose parents say are sleeping through the night are in fact waking up and crying, but are being ignored.

The following table shows the minimum number of night awakenings you might expect at each age; note that babies commonly experience a host of problems that can wake them up more often (as discussed in chapter 6).

Expected Awakenings at Night for Well Babies

From the time baby goes to bed at night to the time baby wakes in the morning—approximately nine to twelve hours

Age	Minimum Number of Awakenings	Main Reasons for Waking Up
0–3 months	2–6	Early sleep is very immature. Infant sleep starts with no definite day-night pattern but with chunks of 3 to 4 hours; it is in the process of consolidating into distinct day and night patterns. The sleep mechanism that enables the brain to transition into sleep is maturing. Hunger/feeding. Babies have small stomachs, and most can't sleep for much longer than 4 hours without a feeding.
3–6 months	0–3	Need help to return to sleep. (Remember that sleep maturity develops at different ages for different babies.) Developmental changes. The brain is changing at a rapid rate—new abilities and feelings can cause a baby to wake. Need comfort or reassurance. Hunger/feeding. Babies still wake up to feed because they are hungry.

Age	Minimum Number of Awakenings	Main Reasons for Waking Up
6–12 months	0–2	Developmental changes, such as crawling and pulling up. Hunger/feeding. Babies can still get hungry in the night, especially when they are having a growth spurt.
9–18 months	0–2	Separation anxiety develops. Babies can now hold images of their parents in their minds, so when they wake up, they may feel anxious because they realize you are somewhere else and not there. Hunger/feeding. Some babies continue to wake for a feed at night.
18 months and up	0–1	Children can wake in the night and seek out their parents up to age 4 or beyond. They usually are just looking for some reassurance that all is okay or want to be close to their parents.

Sources: Beth L. Goodlin-Jones, Melissa M. Burnham, Erika E. Gaylor, and Thomas F. Anders, "Night Waking, Sleep-Wake Organization, and Self-Soothing in the First Year of Life," *Journal of Developmental and Behavioral Pediatrics* 22, no. 4 (2001): 226–233; Sue Sadler, "Sleep: What Is Normal at Six Months," *Professional Care of Mother and Child* 4, no. 6 (1994): 166–167; Patrick McNamara, Jay Belsky, and Pasco Fearon, "Infant Sleep Disorders and Attachment: Sleep Problems in Infants with Insecure-Resistant Versus Insecure-Avoidant Attachments to Mother," *Sleep and Hypnosis* 5, no. 1 (2003): 7–16; Gianluca Ficca, Igino Fagioli, Fiorenza Giganti, and Piero Salzarulo, "Spontaneous Awakenings from Sleep in the First Year of Life," *Early Human Development* 55, no. 3 (1999): 219–228; and Iglowstein et al., "Sleep Duration from Infancy to Adolescence," 302–307.

So when people say "sleeps like a baby," the meaning should be "wakes up a lot" rather than "sleeps solidly and quietly." In the words of child psychotherapist and author Margot Sunderland, "Babies are awful sleepers. When we accept this, maybe we will stop seeing a wakeful baby as some kind of parental failure."[5]

Clearly there is a big difference between what parents are told is normal and what real babies actually do. Most babies who are said to have sleep problems are just doing what babies do; that is, waking up at night and needing help from their parents to get back to sleep.

Reasons That Babies Need Help at Nighttime

Babies and toddlers call for nighttime attention for many reasons. Some reasons apply to all babies, such as the need for feeding, comfort, or reassurance, while other babies have more individual reasons for being wakeful, such as reflux, sleep apnea, food intolerances, or the neurological immaturity of many fussy babies.

Closeness at Night: A Matter of Survival

To understand why babies wake and call for their parents at night, we need to look back in time. A baby born today is biologically and emotionally identical to a baby born in the Stone Age. For much of human history, babies needed to stay close to their mothers to feed, stay warm, and be kept safe from a range of predators, such as wolves, jaguars, lions, and tigers.[6] The extreme vulnerability of babies meant that they simply did not get left alone. Ever! Unless, that is, their parents meant them to die. Sarah Blaffer Hrdy, one of the world's leading social scientists, puts it as follows:

> For more than thirty-five million years, primate infants stayed safe by remaining close to their mothers day and night. To lose touch was death. This explains why, even today, separation from

a familiar caretaker provokes first unease, then desperation, followed by rage and finally despair.

    An infant safe inside a nursery is still well within his or her rights to feel distressed at being left alone. . . . The sensory and cognitive makeup of modern infants, the panic they still feel at separation, is distilled from innumerable past lives in which the infants most likely to survive were those who could prevent separation from their mothers.[7]

Understanding how the nighttime behavior of our children evolved helps us to see their emotional needs with fresh eyes. For a prehistoric baby, making sure a parent was nearby *was* a matter of life and death. For your baby, making sure you are nearby can *feel like* a matter of life and death. The need to know that you will come when called is deeply embedded in your baby's biology (just as the impulse to go to your crying baby is deeply embedded in your biology).[8]

Co-Sleeping—Our Species' Norm

Until recently in the Western world, co-sleeping was often considered to be a somewhat "hippie," if not dangerous, parenting choice. However, attitudes toward co-sleeping are changing, in part due to the fact that so many parents end up co-sleeping because they find it gives them a better night's sleep.

    The work of anthropologist and sleep researcher James J. McKenna has also done a great deal to change opinions on co-sleeping.[9] McKenna presents strong evidence that sleeping close to or with a baby is what humans have always done, and in fact, still do in most cultures today—the main exception being parts of the Western world. McKenna also found that the sleep of babies who are in bed with their mothers is very different from that of babies who sleep alone; their hormonal and sleep processes seem to be regulated by being close to their mothers. They breast-feed more often and experience more REM sleep (see pages 24 to 25 for more information on REM sleep and its importance).

McKenna argues that rather than being a negative or harmful practice, co-sleeping is actually best for babies' development and safety. In fact it could protect babies from sudden infant death syndrome (SIDS) because sleeping close to a parent regulates infants' breathing and keeps them constantly stimulated. McKenna, who is decidedly not a hippie but a very careful research scientist, came to the conclusion that nearly all babies should sleep close to their parents (see pages 113 to 116 for more about co-sleeping and safe bed-sharing guidelines).

And what about those babies who have been sleep trained and no longer call for their parents at night? These babies have learned that their parents won't come to them, but are they scared when they wake up at night? Do they feel frightened and alone in the dark? We don't know for certain—but we think it is highly likely that they do experience these feelings.

The story of Maria, a mother we interviewed in our research, also illustrates how a child can seem to be fine while really feeling quite afraid. Her experience was from when she was about three years old. Maria had very loving parents, but like many parents in the 1970s,

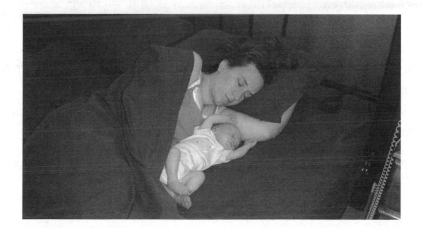

they didn't want children in their bedroom before sunrise—or 7 A.M. to be precise. Every morning for what seemed like months, Maria woke up in the half-light and felt terrified of the shape hanging on the back of her bedroom door—it was actually her brother's robe, but in her mind it was an evil witch who would attack her if she moved. It only became a robe again once it became light enough to see.

Maria never disturbed her parents before 7 A.M., or told them about her fear, but she laid awake frightened for a very long time: outwardly a good sleeper, but inwardly a scared little girl. The point of this story is that the lesson Maria learned was "Don't wake up your parents," not "I can stay asleep all night by myself." A younger child probably won't imagine witches, but could she be lying awake lonely or afraid?

Examining the evolutionary design of babies and young children helps us understand why they might feel frightened at night. It also shows us that while "extinguishing the cries" may bring quiet, it will not soothe or "extinguish" a child's underlying fears or longing for reassurance.

Slow Development of Sleep Skills

Another reason babies need help to get back to sleep at night is because their sleep skills develop slowly. When people talk about *training* or *teaching* a baby to sleep, the impression is that a baby is learning a particular skill, like naming objects (ball, bus, shoes) or tying shoelaces. Yet research about the brain processes involved in sleep suggests that sleep is not a skill that most babies can learn quickly or on their own; they need time and a parent's patient and consistent help for their brains to mature. To explain, let's look at how sleep matures in a healthy normal child.

Children need to develop three sleep abilities: to sleep at night and be awake during the day; to go to sleep without help; and to get back to sleep after waking in the night. To develop these abilities, a number of brain and bodily processes need to mature:

- Ability to distinguish between day and night
- Circadian rhythms
- Quiet and active sleep
- The sleep mechanism

There is no evidence that forcibly interfering with the maturation of these processes is actually desirable; we believe that doing so may in fact set up a person for later sleep problems.

Ability to Distinguish between Day and Night

The majority of babies develop different day-night sleep patterns in the first few months of life, which means they start to do the bulk of their sleeping at night and are more alert and playful during the day. This rhythm is normally established by about three months. Now and then a baby can mix up day and night and may take some gentle encouragement to be less active at night; for example, using dim lighting at sleep time and extra stimulation in the daytime. Thankfully, for anyone who has had a baby who likes night parties, this day/night confusion rarely persists.

Circadian Rhythms

All animals, including humans, contain internal clocks called *circadian rhythms*, which refer to approximately a hundred bodily systems (for example, hormones, temperature, and so on) that go through a daily cycle. When it comes to sleep, the main rhythms relate to light and darkness, body temperature, and stress hormones.

As we noted previously, the brains of most babies sort out the day/ night distinction early on, but the development of the other rhythms is much more variable between children.[10] Individual differences in the rhythm of body temperature and in stress hormone release can account for the differences in wakefulness between babies. For instance, with stress hormone cycles, circadian regulation continues to mature into the third year and at different rates for children.[11] This could explain why some children cannot sleep through the night until older ages. Just as every baby learns to walk and talk at a different rate, so their capacity for putting themselves back to sleep when they wake at night develops quite differently. If you have more than one child, chances are that they will begin sleeping through the night at various ages. For example, Emma, a mother of three, describes the differences between her children's sleep as follows:

Jacinta was able to sleep through the night at six weeks.

Zeb was sleeping through, on and off, from nine months.

Harrison was sleeping through at three and a half years.

Understanding how babies' sleep matures helps us comprehend why most babies are unable to get themselves to sleep and stay asleep for long periods at night.

Quiet Sleep and Active (Rapid Eye Movement/REM) Sleep

Babies have much more rapid eye movement (REM) sleep, also known as *active sleep*, than adults do. REM sleep is the light sleep in which our brains are more active and in which we dream. In contrast to the deep, quiet sleep when your baby is completely zonked, his eyes may flicker and move during REM sleep. It is much easier to wake from REM sleep, which alone explains why babies are more wakeful than adults. REM sleep is also interesting because it seems to have important functions for healthy brain and emotional development.[12]

It is thought that babies experience much more REM sleep than adults because their brains are developing so rapidly.[13] In fact, species such as bottlenose dolphins, who are born very mature, may go through virtually no REM sleep. The more undeveloped a species is at birth—for example, voles and ferrets—the more REM sleep it experiences, and human babies are born less developed than most mammals.

The more immature a species, the more its young need to attach to their caregivers to survive, which means they must develop strong bonds with their parents. The emotional centers of the brain, those that govern love and bonding to our parents, are highly activated during REM sleep.[14] This type of sleep may also, therefore, be important in developing a baby's capacity to love other people.

Recent research on baby sleep shows that how we treat our babies at sleep time can affect their REM sleep.[15] Babies who sleep close to their mothers experience more REM sleep than those who sleep alone.[16] The research into the importance of REM sleep is still in progress, but it does demonstrate another reason why we should view night wakings as a normal, healthy baby behavior. These extra periods of REM sleep during a baby's night sleep are yet another reason for wakefulness.

The Sleep Mechanism

All humans eventually learn to put themselves to sleep without help, although most of us do use some sort of sleep-inducing environment, such as being in a dark bedroom in a nice comfortable bed with pillows. It is also almost impossible to fall asleep if we don't feel safe; for instance, if we hear someone prowling around outside the bedroom.

The shift from being awake to being asleep is governed by what is called the *sleep mechanism*. This mechanism works as a gradual transition in the brain, allowing us to drift out of consciousness. Scientists are still discovering, and arguing about, all the components involved, but to date they have identified up to nine separate stages of brain wave patterns that a brain passes through during the cycle into sleep.[17] At a chemical level, multiple neurotransmitters are released at sleep time, which effectively turn off parts of the brain so our muscles relax and so the brain stops actively engaging with the environment.

Going to sleep should be seen as something like turning a dimmer switch, the slow rotating of which gradually shifts a room from light to darkness. For older children and adults, the complex transition from wakefulness to sleep is something we can do ourselves. Provided there are no sudden noises or lights or disturbing thoughts (Did I lock the door? Did I turn off the stove?), we will drift off to sleep—entering first into the non-REM quiet sleep stage and later moving into dreaming sleep.

The transition to sleep is usually much more difficult for babies because they first enter light, active REM sleep rather than initially moving through quiet sleep. This is why many parents hold their babies for a while until they enter deeper sleep and put them down after fifteen or twenty minutes.

Contrary to popular opinion, humans are not designed to be able to go to sleep without assistance in early life. Transitioning into sleep is rarely something that babies' immature brains can do without some form of help in turning the dimmer switch of the sleep mechanism. For very young babies, this may mean being breast-fed to sleep or being rocked in a parent's arms, while older babies or toddlers may simply need someone to lie with them and stroke their back as they drift off to sleep, and preschool children might be fine with a good-night cuddle and story. We talk a lot more about different settling methods for babies and toddlers in chapter 5.

Physical or Emotional Needs

A whole range of physical problems can contribute to a baby waking up more at night, from teething pain or being overheated to suffering from colic or chronic silent reflux. Some babies just generally require more assistance than others to go to sleep. Emotional challenges can also make a baby anxious and more wakeful; for instance, starting day care, hospital visits, or parental fighting. Unsurprisingly, these problems affect some babies and not others. Many of these issues can be addressed gently, but they should never be addressed by leaving a baby to cry.

Medical Problems

There are many medical problems that disrupt sleep, including general illness and ear infections. In chapter 6, we further address these problems, most of which require professional advice.

High Needs or Heightened Sensitivity

Babies also vary a great deal in the amount of help they need to make the transition to sleep. Anni's first baby, Zac, would lie in her arms, suck his pacifier, and fall asleep while having his forehead stroked. She could even read a novel while putting him to sleep. Upon trying this very appealing sleep technique with her other two babies, she was a bit shocked to find that they would have none of it. In their early months, both Ben and Karl needed a *lot* more movement to help them go to sleep. With these boys, dancing slowly to music or a brisk walk in the baby sling was what they needed.

Some babies are also born more neurologically sensitive than others. These babies have a lower threshold at which they feel stress

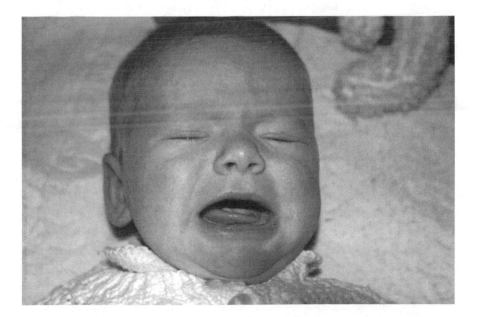

and become upset, and so they tend to cry a great deal.[18] Sensitive babies are really tough for parents to raise, and they are often left to cry alone because people (even many health professionals) really don't understand their true needs. When it comes to sleep, these sensitive babies wake up and cry out more because it takes very little to irritate them; anything—noise, light, and feeling alone or frightened—is likely to cause them to wake. These babies are also much harder to settle for the same reasons: Their brains cause them to feel much more affected by the world, so everything can easily become a bit much to cope with. It is similar to the difference between being in bright sunlight without eye protection as opposed to wearing dark, wide-rimmed sunglasses.

One mother told us of her experience parenting her sensitive child, Dylan:

> My son was not a textbook baby. If there was a how-to manual in utero, my son did not read it. According to the parenting books I read, he would have been classified as a "high-need" baby, except for one major difference. Most books described high-need babies as colicky or generally unhappy—Dylan was not. But maybe that's because I spent nearly every waking, and some sleeping, moment catering to those "high needs" of his. Dylan needed undivided attention and to be held—*all* the time. He was happy as long as he was in my arms, at my breast, or preferably both. No dummy [pacifier], no blankie, no cuddly soft toy for Dylan—my breast was his one and only comfort object.
>
> His penchant for attention and physical contact made sleeping arrangements rather difficult. For a while, we had some success letting him sleep in a vibrating bouncy chair that we left on all night, like a *very* long car ride, but soon he out-grew that. He, unfortunately, was never very fond of his beauti-ful, way-too-expensive cot [crib] that we bought months before he was born. Even when he was beyond the age of needing to breast-feed several times a night (according to the parenting books) he would wake five or six times during the night to do

just that—whether for comfort or food, I was never quite sure. And when he refused to go back to sleep in the cot [crib], I would end up falling asleep holding him in the rocking chair.

I later discovered there may have been more to his behavior than a "high-needs" personality. He had food intolerances that probably contributed to his poor sleeping patterns and his need for physical comforting as well.

Developmental Changes

Many parents are surprised to find that after a period of sleeping through the night, their babies start waking again. Dutch developmental psychologists Hetty van de Rijt and Frans Plooij found that there are approximately ten periods of dramatic change in the brains of children under eighteen months, each accompanied by a clingy period when most babies demand extra attention day and—you guessed it—night. Babies can become restless, refuse to settle, and have difficulty falling or staying asleep. This clinginess and crankiness happens because the babies are bewildered to find that their familiar worlds have turned inside out, and they are bombarded by new perceptions—during these times, the brain can literally be physically restructuring itself. Van de Rijt and Plooij say that during these periods of brain growth, "although to you everything seems the same, to him everything he sees, feels, hears, smells or tastes is somehow different."[19]

These neurological changes may explain why babies sometimes start waking again as they reach developmental milestones. Learning to roll over, crawl, or walk can all mean need for nighttime comfort. We all appreciate our loved ones being extra sensitive and kind when big changes happen in our lives, and babies do too.

When, Oh, When Will My Baby Sleep through the Night?

Some babies are very wakeful at nighttime—and some really do sleep through at six weeks. Parents are rarely offered an accurate explanation as to the reason for this, and they might even come to believe that sleepy babies are good and those who wake up during the night are naughty or manipulative. Scientists are still discovering all the reasons why infants differ so much in their wakefulness, and there are a number of very plausible explanations.

True sleep maturity is something that takes time to develop and occurs at a different rate for each baby. The mysteries of baby sleep are still being uncovered, but what we do know about babies' developing sleep mechanisms should make parents approach sleep training with extreme caution.

Nighttime parenting is simply part of a mom or dad's job description. Some children will continue to wake every so often until school age—even older children and teenagers sometimes need their parents at night when they worry about something. Many problems can also cause babies to wake more often, although these may subside with the right advice.

Key Points

- It is normal for babies to wake up at night. Wakefulness varies from child to child, and it may be affected by the time it takes for the brain's sleep mechanism to mature. Certain problems can also cause some babies to wake up more often.

- Research about the brain processes involved in sleep suggests that it is not a skill that most babies can learn quickly on their own; they need time and a parent's patient and consistent help.

- The research into the importance of REM sleep suggests that we should view night waking as a normal, healthy part of development, and we should approach sleep training—a process that is very stressful for babies—with great caution.

NOTES

1. Thomas Dekker, "Golden Slumbers Kiss Your Eyes," *The Home Book of Verse: American and English, 1580–1918*, ed. Burton Egbert Stevenson (New York: Henry Holt and Company, 1918), 75.

2. Alison Gopnik, Andrew Meltzoff, and Patricia Kuhl, *How Babies Think: The Science of Childhood* (London: Phoenix, 2001), 200.

3. Oskar G. Jenni, Luciano Molinari, Jon A. Caflisch, and Remo H. Largo, "Sleep Duration from Ages 1 to 10 Years: Variability and Stability in Comparison with Growth," *Pediatrics* 120, no. 4 (2007): e769–e776.

4. Beth L. Goodlin-Jones, Melissa M. Burnham, Erika E. Gaylor, and Thomas F. Anders, "Night Waking, Sleep-Wake Organization, and Self-Soothing in the First Year of Life," *Journal of Developmental and Behavioral Pediatrics* 22, no. 4 (2001): 226–233; Melissa M. Burnham, Beth L. Goodlin-Jones, Erika E. Gaylor, and Thomas F. Anders, "Use of Sleep Aids During the First Year of Life," *Pediatrics* 109, no. 4 (2002): 594–601; Sue Sadler, "Sleep: What Is Normal at Six Months," *Professional Care of Mother and Child* 4, no. 6 (1994): 166–167; Patrick McNamara, Jay Belsky, and Pasco Fearon, "Infant Sleep Disorders and Attachment: Sleep Problems in Infants with Insecure-Resistant Versus Insecure-Avoidant Attachments to Mother," *Sleep and Hypnosis* 5, no. 1 (2003): 7–16; and Gianluca Ficca, Igino Fagioli, Fiorenza Giganti, and Piero Salzarulo, "Spontaneous Awakenings from Sleep in the First Year of Life," *Early Human Development* 55, no. 3 (1999): 219–228.

5. Margot Sunderland, *The Science of Parenting: Practical Guidance on Sleep, Crying, Play and Building Emotional Wellbeing for Life* (London: Dorling Kindersley, 2006), 66.

6. Sarah Blaffer Hrdy, *Mother Nature: Maternal Instincts and How They Shape the Human Species* (New York: Ballantine Books, 1999), 411.

7. Hrdy, *Mother Nature*, 97.

8. Jude Cassidy, "The Nature of the Child's Ties," in *Handbook of Attachment: Theory, Research, and Clinical Applications*, eds. Jude Cassidy and Phillip R. Shaver (New York: Guilford Press, 1999), 3–20.

9. James J. McKenna, "Mother-Baby Behavioral Sleep Laboratory at the University of Notre Dame," www.nd.edu/~jmckenn1/lab/faq.html (accessed December 2008); and James J. McKenna and Thomas McDade, "Why Babies Should Never Sleep Alone: A Review of the Co-Sleeping Controversy in Relation to SIDS, Bedsharing and Breast Feeding," *Paediatric Respiratory Reviews* 6, no. 2 (2005): 134–152.

10. Patricio Peirano, Cecilia Algarín, and Ricardo Uauy, "Sleep-Wake States and Their Regulatory Mechanisms throughout Early Human Development," *Journal of Pediatrics* 143, no. 4, suppl. (October 2003): 70–79.

11. Sarah E. Watamura, Bonny Donzella, Darlene A. Kertes, and Megan R. Gunnar, "Developmental Changes in Baseline Cortisol Activity in Early Childhood: Relations with Napping and Effortful Control," *Developmental Psychobiology* 45, no. 3 (2004): 125–133.

12. Gerald A. Marks, James P. Shaffery, Arie Oksenberg, Samuel G. Speciale, and Howard P. Roffwarg, "A Functional Role for REM Sleep in Brain Maturation," *Behavioural Brain Research* 69, nos. 1–2 (July–August 1995): 1–11.

13. Ibid.

14. Patrick McNamara, Jayme Dowdall, and Sanford Auerbach, "REM Sleep, Early Experience, and the Development of Reproductive Strategies," *Human Nature* 13, no. 4 (December 2002): 405–435.

15. James J. McKenna and Sarah S. Mosko, "Sleep and Arousal, Synchrony and Independence, among Mothers and Infants Sleeping Apart and Together (Same Bed): An Experiment in Evolutionary Medicine," *Acta Paediatrica* 83, suppl. 397 (1994): 94–102.

16. McKenna and McDade, "Why Babies Should Never Sleep Alone," 134–152.

17. Robert D. Ogilvie, "The Process of Falling Asleep," *Sleep Medicine Reviews* 5, no. 3 (June 2001): 247–270.

18. Charles A. Nelson and Michelle Bosquet, "Neurobiology of Fetal and Infant Development: Implications for Infant Mental Health," in *Handbook of Infant Mental Health*, 2nd ed., ed. Charles H. Zeanah (New York: Guilford Press, 2000), 37–59.

19. Hetty van de Rijt and Frans X. Plooij, *Why They Cry: Understanding Child Development in the First Year* (London: Thorsons, 1996), 36.

CHAPTER 2

Why Babies Need Their Parents at Sleep Time

*We need to develop the faith that we can
nourish and be nourished by others.[1]*
ROBERT KAREN

*For more than a hundred thousand human generations, our foremothers
cared for their babies in the wild with no crib, carriage or stroller, diapers,
or other accessories, and little clothing. Yet our minimalist forebears thrived
because the mother's body was able to provide all that her baby needed,
and her presence was obviously irreplaceable for infant survival.[2]*
SARAH J. BUCKLEY

We all know what love is—the deep feelings, the swelling heart, the
sense of bonding to another human being. Even though we may not
love our babies straightaway, in time the vast majority of us will feel
an immense love for the little people we created.

What we may not often think about is the difference between
feeling love and *being* loving. They are related, of course; feeling love
usually makes us want to act in loving ways—most of us want to
keep our babies from being hurt, for example. But parents can mis-
takenly believe that they are being loving when they are actually
hurting their children; for instance, by hitting or humiliating them.

Fortunately, there is a science of love. This body of knowledge comes from what is known as *attachment research*, "one of the broadest, most profound and most creative lines of research in developmental psychology."[3] This research explains which parenting behaviors help babies and toddlers feel loved and secure and which do not. It also sheds light on why babies need their parents' assistance to sleep.

What Attachment Research Tells Us about the Care That Babies Need

As we have seen, humans are very immature at birth, as are other mammals, such as monkeys. Biologically, babies need to keep a parent nearby in order to survive, so they are born with an instinctive urge to form a close bond to their parents. This is what is called an *attachment relationship*. It is this innate drive that has kept human babies safe—warm, fed, and protected from threats they are unable to handle—throughout human history. The continual close care of a parent also enables babies to mature into feeling, thinking human beings; our brains and emotions can only develop properly under the careful guidance of another person.

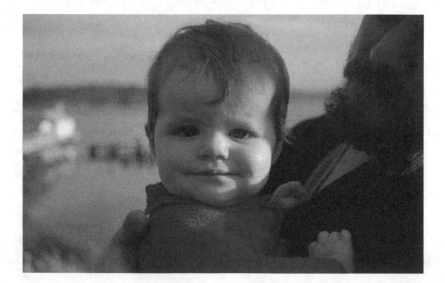

The profound importance of this attachment relationship also explains why babies cry—to let their parents know when something is wrong.[4] If infants become separated from their parents, they need to be able to cry loudly and urgently so their parents hurry back, thereby keeping them safe and maximizing their chances of survival. To babies, having consistent affection, touch, and care is actually as important as food. So when people say in frustration, "My baby is fed, burped, warm, and has a dry diaper—what possible reason does he have to cry?" they are missing their child's number one need: to feel safe by knowing that a parent is close by.

Our babies cannot help but love us. An infant's need to bond with someone, in fact, is so fundamental that he or she will become attached to a poor, or even abusive, caregiver. Even a bad parent is far preferable to no parent, because in evolutionary terms, having no parent meant certain death. Yet the certainty of a baby's love does not mean that the way we parent our children is unimportant far from it. Parenting influences the quality of a child's future relationships, how she copes with life's difficulties,[5] and how her brain is structured (which we discuss in the next chapter). Because babies see themselves as the cause of their experiences, the type of care they receive affects the beliefs they develop about themselves: if their parents are unresponsive, children will see themselves as unlovable and undeserving of comfort.[6]

Mary Ainsworth, a psychologist who is often referred to as the "mother of attachment theory," showed that babies developed either a secure or insecure attachment relationship with their mothers depending on how responsive the mothers were to their needs. Securely attached babies feel confident that Mom and Dad will help them when they need comfort and protection, while insecurely attached babies feel less certain about their parents' availability. Decades of subsequent research have consistently supported Ainsworth's observations; there is a clear connection between responsive parenting and secure attachment.

Secure Attachment Relationships

Around 60 percent of infants are securely attached to their parents.[7] Secure babies are parented in gentle, consistent ways with prompt responses to their cries; the way parents respond is appropriate to what the baby communicates.[8] Parents who consistently tune in and respond to their babies' need for comfort and reassurance teach them to expect that a parent will be available when needed. This expectation allows infants to develop deep trust in their parents. The following is Erika's story:

> I always had trouble sleeping. For a child who can't sleep, it is very lonely and frightening to lie in the dark unable to ask for help. My father told my sister and me that if we were ever frightened or couldn't sleep in the middle of the night to come and wake him up. He said that noses are actually meant to be grabbed as a handle to shake his head and wake him up. I could wake him any time, and he was never angry and never said that he was too tired. Through his reaction, he made me feel that he accepted me with all my faults.
>
> As I grew older, he still supported and assisted me in the same way. I felt that I could go to him with a problem and I wouldn't be judged, just helped. It is rare to find someone who is always there for you, who will support and help and love you unconditionally.

Secure babies know that their parents will be there whenever they're needed. This feeling of security acts like a *psychological immune system*, promoting good mental health and positive self-esteem.[9] Feeling securely loved translates into self-love: "I am lovable; I am worthwhile; I feel good about myself; my feelings are important."

Security also gives babies the confidence to separate from their moms and dads when it is developmentally appropriate and to enjoy their growing independence. It is no surprise, then, that securely attached children do well socially. Their internal confidence and strong sense of self-worth helps them to be likable and easy to get along with. Indeed, secure children are more likely to develop healthy and satisfying relationships with peers and teachers, and they continue to benefit through their teenage years and adulthood.[10] In fact, having a secure attachment relationship is so important for children that the Australian Association for Infant Mental Health encourages parents to make every effort to help their babies feel secure.[11]

Insecure Attachment Relationships and Insecure Feelings

Babies who are repeatedly left to become distressed at sleep time may come to expect (and fear) that their parents will not be available to help them with their difficult feelings, causing them to feel anxious and insecure.[12] In contrast to secure children, insecure children feel less confident that their needs will be met if they openly express them. There are three types of insecure attachment relationships—each of which reflects a different unresponsive parenting pattern.

The most common insecure attachment relationship is *avoidant*. As the name suggests, this attachment pattern reflects the avoidance of emotions. In particular, parents find it difficult to deal with their babies' upset or angry feelings, so they either ignore them or try to stop them from happening. (For example, by saying things like, "Don't you cry now," "Watch that temper," and so on.)

Ambivalent attachment relationships develop when parents are highly inconsistent in their responsiveness to their babies. Infants' cries could be met with anger, no response, or cuddles. This unpredictability is terribly confusing and anxiety-provoking as babies have no way of knowing how their parents will respond.

Disorganized attachment relationships develop when parents consistently hurt or frighten their babies. Babies experience profound distress and confusion: the person who is harming them is also the person to whom they look to protect them from harm.

Children with insecure attachment relationships do not feel confident to express their needs openly to their parents. These children may hide their feelings and seek attention in more subtle manners;

for example, by behaving in negative ways or being overly compliant and helpful.[13]

Insecurity also means children miss out on the development of strong internal regulation—the ability to calm themselves down or seek help when needed. Because they are not consistently helped to calm down, these children do not adequately learn how to regulate themselves and can find it difficult to calm themselves even when comforted. These patterns of attachment relationships are reflected in the brain itself: the neurological systems that enable a person to manage stress are less effectively developed in people who have or had an insecure attachment relationship with their main caregivers (as discussed in chapter 3).[14] Even children who generally feel secure about their parents can have doubts about their trustworthiness and can experience some deeply insecure feelings. For example, a forty-year-old woman said the following:

> I love my parents and we have a great relationship, but there were times as a child when I tried to talk to them about things that upset me and they completely dismissed my concerns. It was clear they were uncomfortable talking about what was worrying me—or thought I shouldn't be upset. Because of this experience, I censor my conversations with them when it comes to certain things—I sometimes say everything is fine even when it is not. I don't trust that they will listen or respond in a way that is helpful.

This knowledge about how insecure attachment relationships develop is important when it comes to thinking about babies and sleep. Those who promote sleep training reassure parents that it doesn't matter if their babies are distressed at sleep time as long as they receive lots of cuddles at other times. Because children can feel insecure when their cries are not regularly met with comfort and soothing, though, this reassurance is profoundly misplaced. By letting babies become distressed at sleep time, parents risk teaching their children that they cannot rely on them to provide soothing and protection when needed.

The two essential messages all children need from their parents are "I am here if you need me," and "You are worth it."[15] Sleep training gives children the message "I am not here," and "You are not worth it."

"Mom and Dad, I Feel . . ."

We have outlined four different types of attachment relationships: secure, insecure avoidant, insecure ambivalent, and insecure disorganized. Secure attachment results from warm and responsive parenting. The other three types are a consequence of various patterns of unresponsive or overtly harmful parenting. One-year-old children with different attachment classifications might say the following if they could talk:[16]

1. *Secure (around 60 percent):* I feel confident that my parents will help me when I'm upset or frightened. If I'm in trouble, I'll ask for help. People can be trusted and relied on. My world feels safe, and I feel lovable.

2. *Insecure Avoidant (around 25 percent):* I have little confidence that my parents will help me when I'm upset or frightened. I deny my needs so I can protect myself from rejection. People are unavailable, so if I'm in trouble, I'll try to manage by myself.

3. *Insecure Ambivalent (around 10 percent):* My parents are unpredictable—sometimes they're loving; other times, they're hostile. Sometimes they help, and sometimes they don't. I don't know what to expect from others, so I feel needy, anxious, and angry.

4. *Insecure Disorganized (up to 10 percent):* My parents may be frightening or seem to be frightened. If I'm in trouble, I know I need them but I'm afraid of them too. I must do my best to control my environment and my relationships.

The Myth That Responding to Babies' Cries Reinforces Bad Behavior

A commonly held belief is that responding to infants' cries will make them cry more. Attachment research contradicts this notion, showing that babies, in fact, cry less in the long term when their parents respond to their cries and signals.

The mistaken belief that responding to babies' cries rewards undesirable behavior has its roots in early psychology. Psychologists in the early twentieth century noticed that actions that were followed by a pleasant experience were likely to be repeated. For example, B. F. Skinner trained pigeons to turn in circles by rewarding them with food. By applying this concept to babies, psychologists theorized that responding to crying would reward this behavior and create "a monstrous crybaby" who would manipulate his parents.[17] Parents were therefore strongly advised to leave their crying babies alone for fear of spoiling them.

Even though these ideas have been resoundingly discredited by research, parents today are still warned not to reward their baby's crying. For example, in *Silent Nights*, Dr. Brian Symon advises mothers as follows:

> Any contact with you is a reward for your child, even if it does not include a feed. It is to your advantage not to reward behaviour that you do not want to see reproduced . . . attending to [your baby] is a reward to crying and will slowly increase the frequency with which that behaviour is exhibited.[18]

And pediatrician Dr. Loren Yamamoto shares similar advice in *Tidbits on Raising Children*:

> Infants are rewarded for crying during the night. Remember the basics of reinforcement. Notice that when a newborn infant cries in the middle of the night, he/she is REWARDED [sic] for

crying by a mother who responds to the crying by carrying the infant (positive reinforcement) and feeding the infant (positive reinforcement). No wonder infants cry a lot at night.[19]

Parents experience terrible heartache as a result of believing that they shouldn't "reward" their babies' crying. "How long do I let my baby cry before I pick her up?" asks the mother of a twelve-day-old girl on an Internet forum. "It's heartbreaking to hear her cry, but I know that if I constantly pick her up when she's upset, she's never going to get into a good groove."

In fact, according to research, babies whose cries are responded to promptly, consistently, and sensitively in their first year are likely to cry *less* frequently than those whose cries are ignored or responded to inconsistently.[20] Over time, babies who are mostly cuddled and comforted when they are upset learn to use means other than crying—such as gestures, facial expressions, and vocalizations—to get their parents' attention. As they grow up, they are more comfortable sharing their feelings with their parents; they trust that their parents will be there to listen to them and take their feelings seriously.

Responding to Babies' Cries Rewards Communication

We believe responding to your baby's crying does not reward bad behavior; instead it rewards *communication*. Learning how to communicate is an important part of a baby's development, and not every baby has the fortitude to continue trying to get a parent's attention when left to cry alone.[21] As psychologist Dr. Zeynep Biringen explains, "If we put off our babies' attempts to get close to us, they will stop seeking us out."[22] Also, infants are so attuned to whether or not their parents are paying attention to their cues or attempts to communicate that they notice—and become upset by—the *emotional* absence of a parent. In what's known as the "still face procedure," psychologists have observed that babies as young as two months old become deeply distressed and disoriented when their mothers suddenly stare at them with blank, expressionless faces.[23]

When this happens, babies try their hardest to get their mothers to respond; for example, by grimacing, frowning, opening their mouths, or gesturing with their arms and legs. Next they develop a somber expression, look away from their mothers, and become intensely sad. They then withdraw into themselves as a way to protect themselves from these difficult feelings. All of this happens in just a matter of minutes. John Bowlby, the founder of attachment theory, observed the following:

> The fact that infants in this situation are so consistently and demonstrably disappointed by the failure in their ability to recapture the mother, and so vulnerable to what they see as her rejection, is evidence of their overriding dependence on a mother's "envelope," on her predictable response to them.[24]

The still face research shows how painful it is for babies to have their communication ignored and be unable to recapture their parent's attention. Mothers, too, find the still face experiment highly distressing.

Babies who can successfully communicate and elicit responses from their parents see themselves as effective; they learn that they can influence their environment and have their needs fulfilled.[25] This mindset is the foundation for independence, good mental health, and a healthy sense of self.

By contrast, babies whose parents don't come to them, no matter how hard they cry, or whose parents are available one minute but absent the next, learn that they are not able to influence the world to meet their needs. Each subsequent loss or disappointment is interpreted as confirmation that they are failures.[26] The feeling of having no control over painful experiences is called *learned helplessness* and has been linked to poor self-esteem, difficulties in relationships, and depression. By going to babies when they call or communicate, you "bequeath the precious gift of optimism to your child."[27]

The Myth That Responding to Babies' Cries Makes Them More Dependent

Many parents are also fearful that responding to crying will make their babies overly dependent on them. This, too, is a myth. In fact, to be effectively independent, children must first be able to depend on their parents for needed comfort and reassurance. According to a group of internationally respected attachment researchers, being sensitive to babies' emotions "serves as the springboard for self-reliance"— they feel confident that they can influence the world to fulfill their needs and achieve their goals.[28]

Just as all babies are born with a drive to attach to a caregiver, they also have an inborn drive for independence.[29] According to Carolyn Quadrio, associate professor of psychiatry at the University of New South Wales:

> It seems that many in our culture fear that without learning as infants to cope without instant comfort we may grow up to be feeble personalities. But other primate infants learn to be independent and to fend for themselves, and their mothers do not try to stifle their instinctive attachment responses. In fact survival of a species is based on this very outcome: the young must learn to fend for themselves, to defend themselves and assert themselves, to fight their own battles, to secure their own food supplies, and to find a mate and reproduce the species. Most species manage this not by stifling instinctive survival mechanisms but by ensuring that these mechanisms are operative. It is curious then that some human cultural groups (including our own) have come to believe that these instinctive survival mechanisms cannot be trusted and should be ignored and suppressed.[30]

Nobody assumes that pushing a newborn in a baby carriage will prevent him from learning to crawl or that holding a ten-month-old's hand as he toddles along will leave him incapable of ever walking by himself. In so many areas of children's development, they are natu-

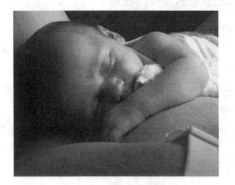

rally dependent on their parents for some time before gradually moving toward independence. This includes sleep. One mother said that one of the most useful pieces of advice she ever received was that "children want to grow up too!"

Far from being unimportant, how parents respond to their babies at sleep time forms part of a pattern of parenting that will affect their entire development. Finding sensitive ways of balancing everybody's need for sleep with babies' need for security is an investment that will pay off for your family for the rest of your lives.

Key Points

- How babies are cared for affects the type of *attachment relationships* they develop with their parents and their feelings about them. Secure attachment relationships and secure feelings help every aspect of children's development and result from parents' consistent sensitivity to their emotional needs—including at sleep time.

- Gently and regularly responding to babies' cries does not reward them for crying or cause them to cry more. Rather, they are rewarded for communicating, and so they gradually learn to cry less often and to use other means of communication instead.

- Your baby will anticipate your behavior, and that of others, based on how you have responded to him in the past.[31] If you are most often responsive, including when he is distressed, he will expect you to be there for him when needed, which will leave him feeling secure.

NOTES

1. Robert Karen, *Becoming Attached: First Relationships and How They Shape Our Capacity to Love* (New York: Oxford University Press, 1994), 4.

2. Sarah J. Buckley, *Gentle Birth, Gentle Mothering* (Berkeley: Celestial Arts, 2009), 220.

3. Jude Cassidy and Phillip R. Shaver, eds., *Handbook of Attachment: Theory, Research, and Clinical Applications* (New York: Guilford Press, 1999), x. The term *attachment research* should not be confused with the term *attachment parenting*, which involves child-lead weaning, co-sleeping, and carrying babies in slings. While all of these are fine parenting practices, they do not guarantee that a child will develop a secure attachment relationship.

4. Jeffry A. Simpson, "Attachment Theory in Modern Evolutionary Perspective," in *Handbook of Attachment*, eds. Cassidy and Shaver, 115–140.

5. Allan N. Schore, *Affect Regulation and the Origin of the Self: The Neurobiology of Emotional Development* (Hillsdale, New Jersey: Lawrence Erlbaum Associates, 1994).

6. Alicia F. Lieberman and Lisa Amaya-Jackson, "Reciprocal Influences of Attachment and Trauma: Using a Dual Lens in the Assessment and Treatment of Infants, Toddlers and Preschoolers," in *Enhancing Early Attachments: Theory, Research, Intervention, and Policy*, eds. Lisa J. Berlin, Yair Ziv, Lisa Amaya-Jackson, and Mark T. Greenberg (New York: Guilford Press, 2005), 100–124.

7. Robyn Dolby, "Overview of Attachment Theory and Consequences for Emotional Development," Child Protection Council, *Seminar 15: Attachment: Children's Emotional Development and the Link with Care and Protection Issues* (1996): 13–24.

8. Jay Belsky, "Interactional and Contextual Determinants of Attachment Security," in *Handbook of Attachment*, eds. Cassidy and Shaver, 249–264.

9. Karlen Lyons-Ruth, Elisa Bronfman, and Gwendolyn Atwood, "A Relational Diathesis Model of Hostile-Helpless States of Mind," in *Attachment*

Disorganization, eds. Judith Solomon and Carol C. George (New York: Guilford Press, 1999), quoted at the Circle of Security Workshop (Parramatta, Australia, March 16–17, 2006), presented by Glen Cooper and organized by the New South Wales Institute of Psychiatry.

10. Nancy S. Weinfield, L. Alan Sroufe, Byron Egeland, and Elizabeth A. Carlson, "The Nature of Individual Differences in Infant-Caregiver Attachment," in *Handbook of Attachment*, eds. Cassidy and Shaver, 68–88.

11. Australian Association for Infant Mental Health, *Position Paper 2: Responding to Babies' Cues* (September 2006), www.aaimhi.org/documents/position%20papers/Position%20Paper%202.pdf (accessed December 2008).

12. Australian Association for Infant Mental Health, *Position Paper 1: Controlled Crying* (Revised March 2004), www.aaimhi.org/documents/position%20papers/controlled_crying.pdf (accessed December 2008).

13. See note 7 above.

14. Omri Gillath, Silvia A. Bunge, Phillip R. Shaver, Carter Wendelken, and Mario Mikulincer, "Attachment-Style Differences in the Ability to Suppress Negative Thoughts: Exploring the Neural Correlates," *NeuroImage* 28, no. 4 (2005): 835–847.

15. Jude Cassidy, "Baby Bonding Video," by Andrea Palpant and David Tanner (North by Northwest Productions, Circle of Security: Early Intervention Program for Parents and Children), www.circleofsecurity.org (accessed October 5, 2006).

16. Public Health Agency of Canada, "Infant Attachment—What Professionals Need to Know," www.phac-aspc.gc.ca/mh-sm/mhp-psm/pub/fc-pc/prof_know-eng.php (accessed October 6, 2006); note 10 above; Karlen Lyons-Ruth and Deborah Jacobvitz, "Attachment Disorganisation: Unresolved Loss, Relational Violence and Lapses in Behavioural and Attentional Strategies," in *Handbook of Attachment*, eds. Cassidy and Shaver, 520–554; note 7 above; and Kristin D. Mickelson, Ronald C. Kessler, and Phillip R. Shaver, "Adult Attachment in a Nationally Representative Sample," *Journal of Personality and Social Psychology* 73, no. 5 (1997): 1092–1106.

17. Karen, *Becoming Attached*, 7.

18. Brian Symon, *Silent Nights: Overcoming Sleep Problems in Babies and Children* (South Melbourne, Australia: Oxford University Press, 1998), 47.

19. Loren G. Yamamoto, *Tidbits on Raising Children: Making Our Most Important Job Easier by Doing It Better*, www.hawaii.edu/medicine/pediatrics/parenting/c05.html (accessed December 2008).

20. Silvia M. Bell and Mary D. Ainsworth, "Infant Crying and Maternal Responsiveness," *Child Development* 43, no. 4 (1972): 1171–1190. Bell and Ainsworth's findings have been replicated by German researchers Karin Grossmann and Klaus E. Grossmann, *Bindungen—Das Gefüge Psychischer Sicherheit (Attachment—The Composition of Psychological Security)* (Stuttgart, Germany: Klett-Cotta, 2004).

21. Stanley Greenspan, with Nancy Breslau Lewis, *Building Healthy Minds: The Six Experiences that Create Intelligence and Emotional Growth in Babies and Young Children* (New York: Perseus, 1999), 99.

22. Zeynep Biringen, *Raising a Secure Child: Creating an Emotional Connection Between You and Your Child* (New York: Berkley Publishing Group/Penguin, 2004), 22.

23. Lynne Murray and Colwyn Trevarthen, "Emotional Regulation of Interactions between Two-Month-Olds and Their Mothers," in *Social Perception in Infants*, eds. Tiffany M. Field and Nathan A. Fox (Norwood, New Jersey: Ablex Publishing Corporation, 1985), 193; and Berry Brazelton and Bertrand Cramer, *The Earliest Relationship: Parents, Infants, and the Drama of Early Attachment* (New York: Perseus, 1990).

24. Brazelton and Cramer, *The Earliest Relationship*, 109.

25. See note 10 above.

26. Mary Dozier, K. Chase Stovall, and Kathleen E. Albus, "Attachment and Psychopathology in Adulthood," in *Handbook of Attachment*, eds. Cassidy and Shaver, 497–519.

27. Greenspan, with Lewis, *Building Healthy Minds*, 95.

28. Weinfield et al., "The Nature of Individual Differences," 78.

29. Jude Cassidy, "The Nature of the Child's Ties," in *Handbook of Attachment*, eds. Cassidy and Shaver, 3–20.

30. Carolyn Quadrio, "Controlled Crying," April 30, 2006.

31. See note 10 above.

CHAPTER 3

Building Your Baby's Brain Day and Night

Human connections create the neural connections from which the mind emerges.[1]
DANIEL J. SIEGEL

It is certainly no accident that the affection most parents feel towards their babies and the kind of attention we most want to shower them with— touching, holding, comforting, rocking, singing, and talking to—provide precisely the best kind of stimulation for their growing brains.[2]
ZERO TO THREE

Parents would never dream of leaving their baby in a room full of toxic fumes that could damage her brain. Yet many parents leave their baby in a state of prolonged, uncomforted distress, not knowing that she is at risk from toxic levels of stress chemicals washing over her brain.[3]
MARGOT SUNDERLAND

Life isn't always easy. We hurt ourselves, a favorite doll breaks, our best friend isn't "best" anymore; in later years, we fail exams, have our hearts broken, work for nasty bosses, and get sick. Yet not everyone experiences these setbacks the same way; some people bounce back from life's many disappointments, while others fret and feel awful, finding it very difficult to calm themselves and feel good again.

Some people have brains that help them manage stress and difficult emotions and feel fine about asking others for assistance. The brains of these people enable them to drive through life's rocky terrain like a well-equipped rally car with a navigator and support team. Other people have brains that are less helpful during challenging times; it's like their brains are set up like an urban sedan—fine for the smooth bits but prone to getting stuck when things get rough. What's more, they usually won't ask the support team for help until it's too late—if ever.

Recent advances in neuroscience, psychiatry, and psychology have shown that the way we are cared for in the first years of life—*including at sleep time*—greatly influences how our brains handle emotions, manage stress, and let us get along with other people.[4] Every person is different, of course, and some babies start out more sensitive than others, but good early care helps us all reach our full potential. In fact, building the brain is a joint construction project between babies and the people who care for them; babies cannot do it on their own. The care of a parent shapes who we are as people—our capacity for joy and excitement; whether we have loving, satisfying relationships or a string of rocky, disappointing ones; how we recover from difficult feelings such as distress and shame; our ability to understand emotions in others and in ourselves; and how we feel about ourselves.

In the previous chapter, we explained why warm, nurturing parenting is so important for emotional development. In this chapter, we look at the neuroscience of love: how sensitive parenting, day and night, creates the biological hardware needed for emotional strength and resilience. We will summarize some of the most interesting findings about how babies' brains work, but we keep the science simple and straightforward. In "Suggested Reading" (pages 197–200), we list several resources and books for those who want to read more about this fascinating field.

The "Unfinished" Baby

Humans might grow up to be the smartest creatures on the planet, but we certainly don't start out that way. As we discussed in previous chapters, human infants are born extremely immature compared to many other mammal babies. In fact, a human baby's brain is only a quarter of the weight of an adult's, with the bulk of our brains being built in a growth spurt over the first two to three years of life. Our brains are not fully developed until we are around twenty years old, and we continue to build new neural connections throughout our adult lives. This length of time is required to enable the brain to develop the complex skills involved in being a human and to adapt to the many different environments in which people live.[5]

The adult human brain is capable of incredible emotional range and highly sophisticated social behavior. But when we are born, our emotional range and social behaviors are very limited; those we do have are designed to maximize our chances of survival.[6] For example, feeding is pleasurable for a baby, while being hungry feels painful, ensuring that a baby will behave in a way to let her parents know when she wants to be fed—making sucking movements with her mouth and eventually crying. Most important, an infant needs to establish a strong bond with her mother and make sure she stays close to her. She can't hang on like a monkey, but if you watch a new baby, you'll see basic social reflexes, such as rooting for the breast, seeking faces, and turning toward a voice—reflexes intended to keep her connected to her parents.[7] And, as we discussed in the previous chapter, if she is left alone, she will usually cry in alarm to bring her mother closer.[8] These basic social behaviors all have a basis in the brain: for instance, if a baby feels threatened by separation from her mother, the *amygdala* is activated, creating the urgent feelings and behaviors that occur in response to danger.[9]

As babies get older, their brains develop further and their emotions become more complex and more uniquely human. The limited range of feelings a baby can experience expands over the first two years of life. Babies start to express happy feelings with those first early smiles around six weeks of age and are soon squealing with joy and delight.[10] When babies are young, they feel no shame, no guilt, no embarrassment—and no pride in what they do well; their brains are simply not developed enough to do so.[11] But these feelings are essential to help people follow the social rules of their culture.[12] And in the second year, these feelings begin to emerge as babies embark on the long process of becoming cooperative social beings.[13]

Emotions are very important. It is also terribly important to be able to regulate emotions—no one wants to be "stuck" feeling a particular emotion or constantly overwhelmed by intense feelings. People need to have the ability to recover from distress, anger, and shame, and avoid becoming completely overexcited when happy. Having an uncontrollable tantrum might be acceptable for a two-year-old—but it's rarely good conduct for grown-ups. However, developing control of emotions, or what is known as "self-regulation," is incredibly complex: Billions of connections need to form between the *limbic system* (the emotional centers of the brain that trigger distress, rage, joy) and the executive higher parts of the brain, located within the *prefrontal cortex*. The strength of these connections governs how well we can regulate our emotions—our capacity to recover from strong feelings and stress and to return to calm.

As the brain grows and matures over time, children develop the capacity to self-regulate and to feel the full range of human emotions. They will be able to feel empathy, express love for others, feel ashamed when they disobey social rules, take pride in their achievements, and figure out what they want and how to get it. New parents will also be relieved to know that children get better and better at controlling their temper, upset feelings, and impulsiveness. However, to develop a brain that is fully emotionally mature takes many, many years—often well past the age of official adulthood.[14] This maturity depends on the strength of the connections between the higher executive

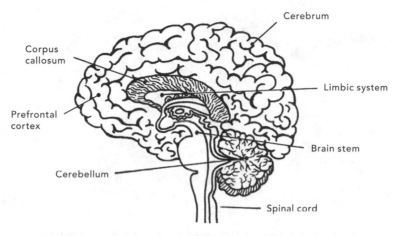

The limbic system (emotional brain) is located beneath the cerebrum (thinking rational brain), which includes the prefrontal cortex.

brain and the emotional brain—and the strength of these connections is highly dependent on a child's parents.[15]

Interactions and Connections

The basic structures of our brains are present at birth: all one hundred billion brain nerve cells (or neurons) are in place. The reason new babies are so neurologically immature is because most of their brain cells are unconnected and therefore unable to communicate with each other. It's like before the Internet existed, when lots of people had computers but couldn't email one another. Neurons need to connect so they can communicate with each other and form the circuitry that enables us to move, see, hear, and talk as well as feel and regulate emotions.

Trillions of brain cell connections are produced in the first years—at a rate of 1.8 million per second between two months' gestation and two years after birth. In fact, nature's superabundant design means babies create far more brain connections than they will ever need. Babies have enormous potential—they can learn any language, grow to love and attach to any parent, and adapt to any human

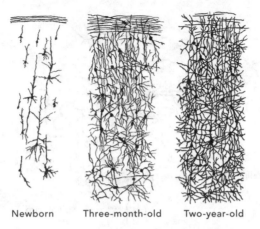

Newborn   Three-month-old   Two-year-old

Difference in extent of brain cell connections between birth and two years.

environment. But clearly people only need to do so much: for example, we don't need to be able to make the sounds of the !Kung people unless we live in the Kalahari Desert. This wonderful brain design enables humans to adapt to the family and society in which they are born. Each baby's brain is molded by their own particular experiences: the connections that they use become amplified and stronger, and those that they don't use wither away.

This phenomenon of culling connections in the brain is called *synaptic pruning*—the brain develops by cutting back, or "pruning," the connections that are not used and keeping those that are. It is similar to shaping an extraordinarily complex hedge—but in this case, what stays and what gets discarded is not up to the gardener but depends on which connections the baby uses. It really is a matter of "use it or lose it." And the more they utilize certain connections, the stronger these connections become.

Strengthening the Emotional Connections between Baby and Parent

The way parents interact with their babies has an enormous influence on how babies' emotional brain pathways develop. What parents *do* greatly affects the strength of the connections that underlie emotional development and self-regulation. This fact is one of the driving motivations for writing this book—to help you understand why and how you are so important to your baby. It is also why neuroscientists who study infants always look at the mother-infant dyad;[16] examining how babies' brains function without their parents or primary caretakers is akin to studying fish behavior out of water. In neuroscientific terms, a baby's main caretaker is known as the "external regulator"[17]—parents are like a fabulous set of training wheels, helping their babies learn to balance on and ride the bicycle of human emotions.

In other words, the brain is literally shaped by the interactions between parents (or other caretakers) and their babies—the smiles and cuddles, the soothing words and gestures, the laughter and tickles, the calming down when they are upset or overexcited. These everyday parenting events are the real brain food, building healthy pathways in an infant's brain. Even just looking lovingly at your baby will cause cells in her brain to start firing and making stronger connections with each other.[18]

As we have seen, the brain pathways that are used the most become strong and powerful as more connections develop. It's a bit like hiking: If one person takes a certain path through the brush, they will make little impact, but if a hundred thousand people walk the same path, it will become a well-worn track. Similarly, if a baby has few experiences of receiving help to calm down when he feels upset, they will have little effect; if he constantly has help to manage his feelings, the establishment of strong pathways in his brain will help him recover from upsetting experiences throughout his life.[19]

Babies' brains don't stop developing in this way when it's time for sleep. Interactions between you and your baby at bedtime will shape your baby's brain just as much as the interactions between you at playtime or any other time. Babies need the experience of feeling safe and nurtured at sleep time so that the brain pathways for healthy emotional development can continue to grow stronger.

Being Attuned to Your Baby

Optimal brain development is not just a matter of parents being physically present—it results from the quality of their interactions with their children. How well parents function as training wheels depends on their attunement to their babies.[20] *Attunement* literally means "in tune"; for example, if you were singing in tune to a song on the radio, you'd be singing the same notes as those coming out of the speakers. Being in tune in parent-baby terms means being in tune emotionally, so that you show your baby that you understand what he or she is feeling; you get in sync, and you react in sync.

Imagine four-month-old Jacob and his mom, Sue Ellen. Sue Ellen is playing with Jacob. She smiles at him and he smiles back. She hides behind her hands, then pops out, and he laughs. She does this again and again—and Jacob laughs each time. The brain processes that allow him to feel joy get a workout—his brain floods with dopamine and opiates, and forges new connections that underlie the experience of happiness.[21] At some point, Jacob will have had enough so he will look away. His brain has become overaroused, and he feels a bit overwhelmed. Sue Ellen, as an attuned mother, stops playing at this point, and waits for Jacob to look back at her and smile before resuming their game. Mothers who are out of attunement might persistently try to stimulate their babies even when they look away, not noticing the signals that they need a break.

When babies are sad or distressed, the role of attuned parents is to comfort them and help them feel all right again, even if this takes some time. This involvement and emotional guidance helps a baby develop strong links between the executive higher brain and the limbic system. Despite what parents are often told, babies can't actually self-soothe when they are upset, because their brains and bodies are simply too immature to do so.[22]

After reading about how we shape our babies' brains, parents might think that they must get it right all the time, that they need to be in sync with their babies at every instant, and that a baby should never be upset. This is absolutely not the case. Misattunement, in itself, is not something to feel guilty about! Mothers and fathers, imperfect beings that we are, often get things wrong and misread our babies, and babies get upset about all sorts of things—things as small as losing eye contact with Mom or as big as a physical injury. These events, often micro-instances, are called *attachment ruptures*, and they happen constantly when parent and baby interact.[23]

What *is* important is that when these ruptures occur, moms and dads regularly help their babies feel okay again, however long it takes.[24] This is called *reattunement*, or interactive repair. For example, it might take Dad a while to notice that his baby is becoming over-stimulated during a game of "this little piggy"—that she is getting too hyped up and there is a crying edge to her laughter. This is fine as long as Dad eventually notices his baby's behavior and checks to see if she needs a rest from the game, a cuddle, or perhaps a nap. These responsive behaviors build the expectation in a baby that "my parents will help me when I'm finding it hard to cope."

This constant cycle of becoming upset and then calming down trains a child's brain pathways to eventually be able to cope well with emotions themselves—just as children are eventually able to ride their bikes without training wheels.

The Stress Response System— Fight or Flight

The *human stress response system* refers to the brain and hormonal systems that help you respond to threats and difficult situations; for example, when you think someone is trying to break into your house, when you're running late to pick up your child, or when you need to meet a deadline—half an hour ago. The stress response system puts your brain on high alert, speeding up your heart rate and sending blood to your muscles and away from your vital organs.

The stress response system evolved at a time when threats to humans were far less complex than they are today, which is why it is known as the fight-or-flight response. Prehistoric threats were of such a nature (for instance, a crocodile or an angry man with a stone ax) that people often had to fight or run away to survive, unlike with a deadline. Even though we don't need to fight or flee in response to many present-day dangers (unless, of course, a wolf does show up in your office), anything our brain perceives to be a threat will still activate the stress response system. People cope with this less-than-perfect system as long as the threats are not too numerous or difficult to overcome and, most important, as long as their stress response system is able to turn itself off when the threat ends.

Luckily, parents can do a lot to help their babies develop healthy stress response systems, which will allow them to weather life's storms. Parents' two main tasks are to protect babies from extreme or chronic stress and to help them calm down when they feel stressed.

Protect Babies from Extreme or Chronic Stress

Babies need to be protected from extremely stressful situations as much as possible. For example, they should not be exposed to violence, neglected, or left repeatedly to cry alone; as a general rule, babies that are crying or fretting are experiencing stress. These situations over-activate the stress pathways in the brain. Repeated experiences of this nature will create a hyperactive stress response system, leaving babies and children far more susceptible to stress later in life and less able to recover from its effects.[25]

Babies also have difficulty coping by themselves with continuous stress of a less extreme nature. Stress hormones in small doses are fine, but they are toxic for our brains and bodies when exposure becomes chronic. We don't know how much stress babies can safely manage on their own (that is, how frequently they can be left to cry without comfort before the brain is affected). Research shows that chronic exposure to stress hormones literally shrivels parts of the brain, particularly those that govern short-term memory.[26] Continual exposure to stress can also make babies, children, and adults hypersensitive so that they are constantly in a state of high alert. Children in this state find it hard to learn, and their behavior tends to be either aggressive or withdrawn.[27]

Help Babies Calm Down When They Feel Stressed

Parents can actively assist the development of the stress response system by helping babies calm down when they feel stressed.[28] This means reassuring or comforting your baby when she is upset, perhaps with an affectionate look and a smile or by cuddling, patting, or breast-feeding: whatever will help your baby feel okay again.

These responsive parenting behaviors are the same as those that promote attachment security, which we discussed in chapter 2. Securely attached children and adults have superior internal mechanisms to calm themselves down when they become anxious.[29] Their strong executive brain function sends effective messages to turn off the stress response, and they have more recep-

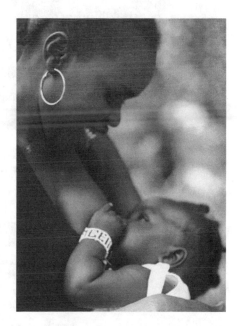

tors in their brains to absorb stress chemicals.[30] They are also far more able to seek help from others when they need it because the thought of receiving assistance or support doesn't make them feel more anxious. This resilience results from the parenting they received, which enabled the optimum development of their stress response systems. So, in the words of neuroscientist Allan N. Schore, "Resilience in the face of stress is an ultimate indicator of attachment security."[31]

What You Can and Can't Control

Some babies are exposed to extreme stress over which their parents have no control. They may have been born prematurely or may have underwent painful medical procedures; they may have been in a serious accident or may be grieving the loss of a parent. Although you can't change what happened, you do have control over how you respond to your child. Responsive care, lots of cuddling, and sensitive play will stimulate your baby's brain to release hormones that help him feel good and alleviate the effects of these stressors on his developing stress response system.

The best thing for babies' stress response systems is not to leave them alone when they cry, but rather to gently hold and soothe them. Try to stay calm. It is more helpful to think "I can be here for my baby" than "I must stop the crying." When children are crying in your arms, they can feel, smell, and see you—just your presence is enormously comforting, even if the crying continues. Holding your babies causes their brains to release chemicals that help reduce feelings of stress. Think about the difference between sobbing your heart out all alone or sobbing your heart out with someone you love holding you or sitting with you.

Sometimes, however, your baby won't stop crying no matter what you do. If you have a colicky baby, this may happen daily. Anni's baby Ben would start crying about 4 P.M. every day and would not settle down until late evening. Professionals sometimes advise parents to let their babies cry alone in such instances, but this is poor advice because it creates another layer of distress for babies; they now have to cope with being left alone in addition to whatever else is upsetting them. (Of course, if you feel so overwhelmed by constant crying that you fear you might hurt your baby, it is best to leave the child alone while you take time to recover.) We discuss some ideas for dealing with colic in chapter 6 (see pages 137 to 138).

Some babies with vulnerable dispositions need extra help to calm down when they feel stressed; they are ill-equipped to deal with even low levels of stress by themselves, the kinds of experiences that more robust babies handle easily. These babies may have been born very sensitive, or they may become sensitive due to difficulties after birth. Those who may be vulnerable include the following:

1. *Babies who are adopted or foster children:* Adopted and foster children often experience neglectful, abusive, or disruptive care before they are placed with their new parents. This means that they are particularly sensitive to stress because they most likely missed out on the consistent nurturing that is necessary for healthy brain development. They may have lost a parent or been in numerous foster care homes, and they are likely to feel frightened and overwhelmed. It is important to give these babies responsive, nurturing parenting so they can develop trust in their new caretakers and feel secure in their new families.

2. *Babies who are born prematurely:* Premature babies need extra care because they are more immature at birth than full-term babies. This means that their brain development starts behind that of full-term babies, making them far more sensitive to the impact of stressful events.[32] For many premature babies, their early weeks and months include numerous medical interventions and lengthy separations from their parents. "Kangaroo care," in which a baby is held next to his mother's skin for prolonged periods of time, has been found to be very helpful for premature babies, promoting growth and development and reducing stress and crying.[33]

3. *Babies who experience physical or psychological trauma:* Babies who experience trauma of some sort, perhaps due to abuse or neglect or invasive medical procedures, are also more sensitive. These babies are easily overwhelmed by their environments and they may be very fearful. Like other babies who have difficult starts, they particularly need parenting that responds to their extra emotional needs.

4. *Fussy or high-need babies:* Some babies are just born more neurologically immature and sensitive. These babies are often termed *colicky*, *fussy*, or *high-need*, and they are much more easily distressed than less sensitive babies.

All of these babies are also more likely to be wakeful at night and to have problems settling to sleep. They need extra-sensitive, responsive, and patient parenting—this kind of love and care gives them the best chance to thrive.

Helping build babies' brains is the most important job parents have; thankfully, it is also the most pleasurable, because the brain is literally constructed with loving interactions. Leaving babies to cope with stressful situations alone won't toughen them up or teach them to be independent. Infants' brains are exquisitely designed to develop under the guidance of an adult brain; all of their senses need to be anchored to this brain. Keeping this anchor steady allows your baby's brain to forge the pathways needed to become a happy, loving, and resilient adult.

Key Points

- Babies' brains develop as a result of their relationship with their parents. Babies need the experience of feeling safe and nurtured at all times, including sleep time, so the regulatory pathways in their brain can grow stronger.

- Babies rely on their parents to regulate their emotions. They are not equipped to deal with stress by themselves.

- Responsive care fosters a secure attachment to a caregiver, which is evident in the structures of babies' brains. This security enables children to deal effectively with stress as they grow up.

NOTES

1. Daniel J. Siegel, "Toward an Interpersonal Neurobiology of the Developing Mind: Attachment Relationships, 'Mindsight,' and Neural Intergration," *Infant Mental Health Journal* 22, nos. 1–2 (2001): 72.

2. Zero to Three: The Nation's Leading Resource in the First Years of Life, "Brain Development," www.zerotothree.org/site/PageServer?pagename =ter_key_brainFAQ (accessed October 2006).

3. Margot Sunderland, *The Science of Parenting: Practical Guidance on Sleep, Crying, Play and Building Emotional Wellbeing for Life* (London: Dorling Kindersley, 2006), 40.

4. Allan N. Schore, "Effects of a Secure Attachment Relationship on Right Brain Development, Affect Regulation and Infant Mental Health," *Infant Mental Health Journal* 22, nos. 1–2 (2001): 7–66; and Megan R. Gunnar and Carol L. Cheatham, "Brain and Behaviour Interface: Stress and the Developing Brain," *Infant Mental Health Journal* 24, no. 3 (2003): 195–211.

5. Zero to Three: The Nation's Leading Resource in the First Years of Life, www.zerotothree.org/site/PageServer?pagename=key_brain (accessed May 2007).

6. Jaak Panksepp, "The Long-Term Psychobiological Consequences of Infant Emotions: Prescriptions for the Twenty-First Century," *Infant Mental Health Journal* 22, nos. 1–2 (2001): 132–173.

7. Louis Cozolino, *The Neuroscience of Psychotherapy: Building and Rebuilding the Human Brain* (New York: W. W. Norton & Company, 2002), 173.

8. Jude Cassidy, "The Nature of the Child's Ties," in *Handbook of Attachment: Theory, Research, and Clinical Applications*, eds. Jude Cassidy and Phillip R. Shaver (New York: Guilford Press, 1999), 3–20.

9. Cozolino, *The Neuroscience of Psychotherapy*, 242–245.

10. Jennifer M. Jenkins, Keith Oatley, and Nancy Stein, *Human Emotions: A Reader* (Cambridge: Cambridge University Press, 1998).

11. Allan N. Schore, *Affect Regulation and the Origin of the Self: The Neurobiology of Emotional Development* (Hillsdale, New Jersey: Lawrence Erlbaum Associates, 1994).

12. Dirk Fabricius, "Guilt, Shame, Disobedience: Social Regulatory Mechanisms and the 'Inner Normative System,'" *Psychoanalytic Inquiry* 24 (2004): 309–327.

13. Cozolino, *The Neuroscience of Psychotherapy*.

14. Elizabeth R. Sowell, Bradley S. Peterson, Paul M. Thompson, Suzanne E. Welcome, Amy L. Henkenius, and Arthur W. Toga, "Mapping Cortical Change across the Human Life Span," *Nature Neuroscience* 6, no. 3 (2003): 309–315.

15. Allan N. Schore, *Affect Dysregulation and Disorders of the Self* (New York: W. W. Norton & Company, 2003).

16. See note 11 above.

17. Schore, "Effects of a Secure Attachment Relationship," 7–66.

18. Schore, *Affect Regulation and the Origin of the Self*, 76.

19. Cozolino, *The Neuroscience of Psychotherapy*, 33.

20. Maria Legerstee, Gabriela Markova, and Tamara Fisher, "The Role of Maternal Affect Attunement in Dyadic and Triadic Communication," *Infant Behavior and Development* 30, no. 2 (2007): 296–306.

21. Schore, *Affect Dysregulation and Disorders of the Self*, 147.

22. Sunderland, *The Science of Parenting*, 79.

23. See note 17 above.

24. See note 17 above.

25. National Scientific Council on the Developing Child, "Excessive Stress Disrupts the Architecture of the Developing Brain," 2005, www.developingchild.net/reports.shtml (accessed March 2, 2006).

26. Cozolino, *The Neuroscience of Psychotherapy*, 25–26

27. Megan R. Gunnar and Ronald G. Barr, "Stress, Early Brain Development, and Behaviour," *Infants and Young Children* 11, no. 1 (1998): 1–14.

28. See note 17 above.

29. Allan N. Schore, "Attachment, Affect Regulation, and the Developing Right Brain: Linking Developmental Neuro-science to Pediatrics," *Pediatrics in Review* 26, no. 6 (2005): 204–217; and Gunnar and Cheatham, "Brain and Behaviour Interface," 195–211.

30. Sue Gerhardt, *Why Love Matters: How Affection Shapes a Baby's Brain* (East Sussex, England: Brunner-Routledge, 2004), 66.

31. Gerhardt, *Why Love Matters*, 207.

32. Dianne Maroney, "Recognizing the Potential Effect of Stress and Trauma on Premature Infants in the NICU: How Are Outcomes Affected?" *Journal of Perinatology* 23, no. 8 (2003): 679–683.

33. "Kangaroo Mother Care," www.kangaroomothercare.com (accessed October 2007).

CHAPTER 4

Why Sleep Training Is Bad Advice

An error does not become truth by reason of multiplied propagation,
nor does truth become error because nobody sees it.[1]
MAHATMA GANDHI

Now that we recognize how important feeling loved and secure is for babies, we can understand that how we put them to sleep matters greatly. Before we discuss gentle bedtime methods (which we do in part 2), however, we'll take a closer look at sleep training—also known by a host of other names, such as "cry it out" or the Ferber Method—the most common advice parents receive about helping their babies sleep. Sleep training programs, at their core, instruct parents to "train" their babies to fall asleep on their own by letting them cry for a certain amount of time before offering any comfort. This chapter explores sleep training, how it affects babies and parents, and just why it is such bad advice.

What Is Sleep Training?

The main goal of sleep training is to teach babies to go to sleep without help (such as rocking or feeding) or aids (such as pacifiers). Babies are said to need sleep training if their parents are unhappy with the way they sleep—or if the way they sleep doesn't meet certain expectations. Parents may use sleep training if they are worried babies cannot go to sleep by themselves, do not sleep through the night, or do not take naps often enough or for long enough. Success is declared when babies fall asleep without their parents nearby and when they can go back to sleep without help when they wake up at night.

Sleep training is not a modern concept. Its origins lie in nineteenth-century attitudes toward children, when people started applying the notions of good science and hygiene to the complex world of parenting. Luther Holt, a popular doctor considered to be a child care expert at the time, thought parents should train their children out of bad habits and that they shouldn't be too affectionate. He insisted that parents avoid closeness with their children and not pick them up when they cried, sternly advising against affectionate contact such as rocking.[2] Later, John B. Watson, president of the American Psychological Association, continued this campaign against affection. "Mother love is a dangerous instrument," he warned and noted that picking up crying children or feeding children according to their needs were indulgences that would harm them.[3]

While child development experts have moved away from these antiquated theories, the advice to withhold parental love and affection is unfortunately still the essential ingredient of sleep training. Today sleep training instructions can be found in parenting books, magazines, and newspapers, and on television, the radio, and the Internet. Consider the advice offered by these contemporary baby sleep authors: In an article in *Practical Parenting* magazine, Tizzie Hall recommends, "Let baby know . . . that no matter how much shouting [crying] takes place you will not be coming in until he's asleep. . . . You must be strong and determined if you want to win this argument."[4] Dr. Brian Symon, in *Silent Nights: Overcoming Sleep Problems in Babies and Children*, tells parents that "the overtired baby is very easy to treat. Unfortunately few treatments are so difficult to carry out. . . . The treatment is do nothing . . . put your hands in your pocket and walk away."[5] And in *Teach Your Baby to Sleep through the Night*, Charles Schaefer and Michael Petronko write that parents must "be absolutely consistent in adhering to the procedures. Don't give in—no matter how much your baby cries."[6]

Some health professionals insist that it is essential for children's development to learn how to sleep independently, warning of terrible health and developmental consequences if they do not. Others simply say that sleep training is a valid choice for parents. Each sleep training program varies slightly, but most have common elements, which we discuss below.

"Guaranteed Success" if You Stick with the Program

Parents are told that sleep training can easily modify their baby's sleep. They are usually advised to stick with the program, no matter what. For example, sleep specialist Dr. Richard Ferber gives parents the following advice in his popular parenting guide: "You should follow the schedule consistently. Your child must learn what to expect. If you are lenient sometimes and firm others, your child will always assume that this may be one of the times you are going to give in."[7] Similarly, pediatrician Dr. Christopher Green suggests, "Never back off, and hard as it may be in the early days, don't give up. . . . Keep this routine going tonight, tomorrow and for as long as it takes to work. Don't give an inch whatever you do."[8]

Withholding Comfort

All programs advise parents to put babies in their cribs awake so they can learn to go to sleep by themselves. Some recommend leaving babies to cry it out until they fall asleep, without returning at all to check on them or console them. Although these techniques can change their sleep behavior, they clearly cause many babies immense distress, as we'll see later in this chapter. Other programs counsel parents to return to their babies after a set period of time to offer brief reassurance (for example, a minute or two of patting) and then leave their babies again for fixed (and usually increasing) periods of time before offering brief comfort again. An example of this type of program recommends waiting for the child to cry for two minutes before providing comfort, then four, then six, then eight and then ten, going to the child every ten minutes after that.[9] Parents are generally advised to limit the comfort they offer when they return and to leave their babies in their cribs, not to pick them up or make eye contact— just pat the baby's bottom or stroke the baby's head.

Although these programs may sound gentler than the cry-it-out method, many parents don't find this to be the case. One parent said,

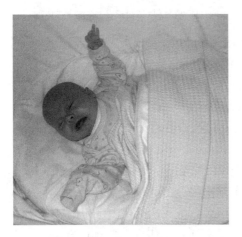

"To listen to your baby scream, even for just two minutes, and then have that stretch out to nine before you're 'allowed' to go in, is emotionally devastating. Do that for over an hour every time he's meant to have a nap, and it seems like your whole day is taken up listening to him cry." See later in this chapter for more about parents' experiences with sleep training.

Specific Age Recommendations

Most programs advocate a specific age by which parents should "train" their babies to sleep. The recommended age to commence sleep training varies: Some programs advise leaving babies to cry alone from shortly after birth.[10] Others suggest waiting until a baby is four or six months old. Modified versions based on the same principle— teaching independent sleep by leaving children for extended periods of time—are available for toddlers. Parents who want to sleep train their toddlers are often advised to stop their children from leaving their rooms at bedtime or nap time. Suggested methods include shutting the door,[11] removing the door knob and fastening the door shut,[12] installing a latch lock,[13] or keeping the door slightly ajar by installing a burglar lock with a chain.[14]

Repeating the Program

Parents who have "successfully" sleep trained are told to expect that their child may begin to call for them again at night (for example, after teething, illness, or a vacation). When this occurs, parents are encouraged to repeat sleep training as soon as possible. It is not uncommon for parents to redo sleep training frequently over the first few years of their child's life. One parent explains, "I didn't know ahead of time is that it is not a 'once and for all' kind of thing. We had to do a little 'refresher course' after traveling, illness, and the like."

Using the Program Day and Night

Sleep training is usually recommended for both daytime naps and nighttime sleep, although some parents only use it at night.

Can Babies Really Self-Soothe?

One reason that parents are advised to use sleep training is to teach their babies to self-soothe. It is suggested that leaving babies to cry themselves to sleep will teach them to calm themselves when upset. However, the brain structures that enable people to calm themselves when stressed (in particular, the orbitofrontal cortex) do not fully mature for years.

Throughout the preschool years and beyond, children often need their parents to help them feel right again when they are upset, angry, or ashamed. They feel abandoned and distressed if forced to endure long periods of disconnection from a caregiver.[15] According to psychiatrist and associate professor Daniel J. Siegel, "As the child's brain matures into the preschool years, the emergence of increasingly complex layers of self-regulation becomes possible."[16] As one mother observed, "I doubt that a baby who can't even control his bowels is capable of controlling his emotions."

Babies who stop crying after being left alone when distressed haven't learned to self-soothe because they lack the brain mechanisms to do so; rather, they have learned to give up crying for help.

Is Sleep Training Safe?

At the heart of all sleep training programs is the promise that parents and their babies will soon be well rested and much happier, so it is no wonder that it seems like an inviting option. Even so, many parents feel hesitant about these techniques, expressing concern that sleep training will emotionally damage their babies. Given that a host of professionals recommend sleep training, we assumed we would find a strong body of research to support its safety. We looked for evidence that sleep training was safe for babies and that it did *not* contribute to the following:

- Highly elevated stress levels—during sleep training and subsequently at sleep onset (even if the baby is not crying)
- Changes to neural systems underlying emotional regulation
- Changes to sleep architecture (altering the proportions of REM and non-REM sleep)
- Increased feelings of insecurity about parents' availability and reliability

We found that most research on sleep training shows that it "works" in the short term for many babies; that is, it stops them from crying out for their parents.[17] Research also shows that parents often feel better when their babies don't wake up at night.[18] But as far as reassuring parents that sleep training is safe for their babies, we could find no credible research. There is neither research examining babies' stress levels after being left to cry themselves to sleep nor research assessing whether sleep training affects babies' neurological capacity to regulate emotion (for example, to calm down after being upset).

On the other hand, we did find research that shows sleep training reduces REM sleep.[19] Given the importance of REM sleep for brain development (see pages 24 to 25), this research seems to prove the method's potential to impede proper development.

A number of studies claim to show that sleep training has a positive impact on the behavior of children and appears to contribute to feelings of security.[20] But as we explain in chapter 2, a child's apparently calm behavior does not in itself indicate secure feelings. For example, the "good" children who are quiet and seemingly cooperative—but do not always trust their parents to respond well if something worries them—are not necessarily "secure" children. Perhaps more troubling, however, is that all of these studies examine only short-term impact; most involve small numbers of children; and none utilize internationally recognized tools for assessing emotional security.[21] In fact, most use parental self-reports as their main methodology for assessing a child's feelings of security, leaving wide open the possibility of biased reporting, because parental expectations may color the results. The largest study, involving ninety-five children, employs a technique to measure feelings of security that even the author describes as "very subjective" and of "unknown and probably low validity and reliability," limited by a "lack of direct observation of child behaviour and parent child interactions."[22]

So, at this stage, the research into sleep training's effect on babies and young children is still a long way from reassuring parents that it is beneficial or safe, especially in the long term. In spite of this, many professionals continue to assure them that there is no evidence that sleep training does any harm.

Will Sleep Training Harm Older Babies and Toddlers?

Many professionals do not recommend sleep training for babies under six months but tell parents that it is safe after that age. From examining the way the brain develops, we believe that there is no safe age for sleep training.

For newborns or babies a few months old, the brain's response to being left to cry alone is deep fear, distress, and rage. Repeated experiences of this kind in infancy can imprint on the brain's primitive structures, and these emotions can become a core part of a person's personality. For instance, as this person grows up, he or she may experience persistent inexplicable fear or become intensely enraged at the slightest provocation.

At about eight or nine months to about sixteen months of age, a baby's brain goes through *attachment-driven right brain growth*: a surge occurs in the parts of the brain that start enabling babies to regulate their own emotions. For these parts of the brain to develop in a healthy way, babies need their parents to help them manage difficult feelings; they are in no way ready to do this by themselves—and will not be for many years. It is at this time, too, that babies begin to exhibit fear of strangers and separation anxiety, and so they can be expected to protest most fiercely at sleep training—they are letting Mom and Dad know that their brains still very much need their presence.

At around fifteen or sixteen months, children start to develop the capacity to feel shame. This is an incredibly strong emotion and can occur when parents emotionally withdraw from their toddlers, as they do in sleep training. Child psychiatrist Daniel J. Siegel and early childhood expert Mary Hartzell put it this way: "For any of us, not having connection when we need it can induce intense emotion. That emotion is shame. . . . Prolonged disconnection [from a parent] can create shame and humiliation that is toxic for the child's growing sense of self."[23]

As with all difficult emotions, children need help to recover from shameful feelings. They should never be put in situations in which they feel excessive shame and have to try to manage it alone. Leaving children in states of prolonged, unregulated shame may make it more difficult for them to deal with shame as adults; for example, they may become very easily shamed or struggle to bounce back from the sick feelings that shame engenders.

Sleep Training Can Create Physical Risks

Asking parents to disregard their babies' cries also sets up a dangerous situation in which a child in serious physical trouble could be ignored. For example, parents who watch the clock as their babies cry may not come running in to respond to a physical emergency—children can fall out of cribs, catch a limb in the bars of the crib, or choke on their vomit. Such risks are sometimes readily apparent in parents' descriptions of sleep training:

> At one point, our son started choking! Thank God we were right there and helped him unblock his passages. What if we had not been so attentive?

> [My son] rolls over and gets his arms and legs stuck in between the bars of the cot [crib], and I am worried that if he starts to get tired while still facedown, he will suffocate himself. . . . He always ends up hitting his head, getting stuck facedown, or hurting an arm or leg between the bars.

These examples illustrate that sleep training risks not only a baby's psychological well-being but can also create situations of serious physical danger—especially if parents are completely "deaf" to their baby's distress.

Why Do Experts Recommend Sleep Training if It Isn't Safe?

According to child mental health specialist Bert Powell, "we know more about children and development than at any time in history, and yet there is a huge gap between what is known and what is practiced in our culture."[24] Many professionals such as pediatricians, nurses, and midwives continue to recommend sleep training for many reasons, including the following:

- *Lack of knowledge on the subject:* Many don't receive formal training on the nature of normal infant sleep and may not have the opportunity to consider the implications of recent psychological and neuroscience research.

- *Subjectivity to cultural misconceptions:* Doctors and other health-care professionals are as susceptible as any other person to cultural myths; for example, that crying babies will be spoiled if they're picked up and cuddled or that babies should sleep through the night at an early age.

- *Personal experience and bias:* Some may be influenced by their own childhood experiences. For instance, a pediatrician whose feelings were dismissed as a child may be more likely to counsel parents to disregard their children's feelings rather than one whose feelings were responded to in a sensitive manner.[25]

- *Unsupportive work environment:* Some may not receive adequate emotional support from their colleagues and workplace, and so may psychologically shut down from their patients' distress to survive their work environment. It's difficult working with exhausted parents and babies, and the ability to offer a concrete, simple solution feels good.

- *Unawareness of alternative approaches:* Many may not be aware that there is a range of gentle methods available to modify babies' sleep habits. As one nurse said to Beth, "If not controlled crying, then what?"

While these experts may know many things about babies, it seems they are unfamiliar with the research that shows babies feel safe, secure, and loved when someone responds promptly and consistently to their cries. They also seem unaware that sleep training has many downsides for both babies and their parents.

Is Sleep Training Stressful for Babies and Parents?

Parents are often told that sleep training involves only a few nights of crying. In reality, it is rarely a brief, stress-free event. Babies and young children may be extremely distressed for long periods over several nights. Some authors suggest that returning briefly to comfort them before leaving again is kinder than letting them cry it out; however, both techniques can cause great emotional pain.

Crying without Comfort Distresses Babies

While we may *think* that five or ten minutes of crying are insignificant, it certainly doesn't *feel* insignificant to many babies and parents. Young children experience time subjectively, and their distress can seem to last forever to them, even if only a short period of time passes on the clock.[26] Babies don't generally stop crying after only a few minutes of sleep training. In fact, they often cry for hours at a time. One mother told us, "It was at least three weeks of an hour or two of crying each night before he slept through the night." Some parents follow advice to routinely leave their babies to cry to sleep soon after birth and rarely attend to them at bedtime. Other parents commence sleep training when their babies are a few months old. Either way, many children endure the stress of sleep training for weeks or even months. Having been promised that the program will work if they persist, parents often see no option but to leave their babies to scream for hours at a time, day after day, week after week. One parent recounted to us, "I was told it would take three days, but it took three weeks."

Sleep training doesn't always work as experts say it will, so babies continue to cry at bedtime and when they wake up. In some cases, long after the first few nights and weeks have passed, babies are still crying themselves to sleep. One woman told us that her friend "has been using [sleep training] for about a year, and her child still cries herself to sleep."

In short, countless children are being left to cry alone for *tens, if not hundreds*, of hours before their third birthday arrives. This is real emotional suffering and stress endured by vulnerable infants and toddlers who are powerless to understand what is happening to them.

Babies Can Become Sick from Crying and Stress

Concerned parents are often advised not to worry about the extreme distress brought about by sleep training—and told that it won't harm their babies. Recent advances in neurological research reveal that in fact, parents are correct to be worried. Being left to cry causes acute anguish and deep terror for some babies, who experience stress so intense that it overwhelms their ability to cope. They may rage and scream hysterically; they may become so upset that they vomit, literally sickened by stress. That type of response has all the hallmarks of trauma.

Babies can experience being left to cry alone as life-threatening; they can feel utterly and completely helpless. For many people, this is hard to understand: How can a baby feel terrified in a safe bedroom and crib? The following are the words of one dad:

> We let her cry herself to sleep in the crib. It's painful to listen to at first, but after a couple of days you get used to it, and after a week or so, it actually becomes pretty hilarious. All you are doing is gently laying her down in a nice, warm baby-sized sleep space and she's screaming like a cat being butchered. I understand it's going to be even funnier when language is thrown into the mix and she starts screaming "Help me! Save me!" in these benign situations.

What this father didn't comprehend is that being left alone can *feel like* a dramatic threat to babies. In chapter 1, we discussed how there was a time in human evolution when not having a parent nearby meant death—from exposure, cold, or predators. Human evolution explains why babies become so angry and upset when left by themselves; they may literally fear for their lives.

As we noted earlier, sleep training can result in babies crying so hard that they vomit. Nausea is a well-recognized response to psychological trauma, when a person is extremely stressed, the body releases a hormone known as *vasopressin* that can affect the gut in such a way that it makes a person feel sick.[27] This explains why many babies—approximately one in five—will vomit as a result of the sleep training process.[28]

Baby sleep authors and other health professionals often warn parents not to allow the vomiting to disrupt sleep training, to clean it up in a no-nonsense way, and then leave the baby to continue crying. Behind this advice is the idea that consoling babies who throw up will teach them to do so on purpose in order to receive the attention they desire. Jean Kunhardt, a child sleep specialist, offers the following observation to parents:

> If during [the first] few days [of sleep training] your child did not learn that throwing up can get him what he wants, he will not begin to use it as a method of keeping his parents captive.[29]

Sadly, some parents also view vomiting as a sign of manipulation. A mother shared the following on an Internet forum:

Renata went through a phase of crying so much that she gagged and vomited badly. Once she realized that this got her the attention she needed so much, she started doing it on purpose. As soon as we took her into her room, she would gag a little to try to make herself sick. This was extremely upsetting and disturbing! We had to ignore her vomiting and clean her up quickly and get her back into bed. She soon learned that it was getting her nowhere.

These interpretations of vomiting incorrectly assume that babies are cognitively sophisticated enough to be able to manipulate their parents in such a way. Even if babies *were* vomiting to get their parents' attention, it is astounding that anyone could think it was okay for babies to feel they have to take such drastic measures to get the comfort they need.

While the overwhelming distress caused by sleep training can make some babies throw up, the memory of trauma can also elicit nausea. If babies are distressed to the point of vomiting during sleep training, each time they are placed in that situation (for example, in their cribs alone and crying), the brain's fear center (the *amygdala*) is reactivated, stress hormones surge, and they feel nauseated. Babies who vomit during sleep training are not being difficult or manipulative—they are experiencing immense emotional pain and desperately need their parents.

Effect of Early Trauma on Adults

According to psychiatrist Dr. Isla Lonie, "In therapies with people who come because they keep 'losing it,' we often find that there has been some form of early trauma [that] occurred before there was speech to be able to think about it, and so to manage the [traumatic] event at an intellectual level.[30] Good evidence is emerging that situations of stress in infancy cause damage to important nerve tracts in the brain."[31]

Brief Comfort Is Not Comforting

Proponents of sleep training usually advise parents to offer comfort at intervals, to go to their babies and briefly pat or stroke them. This is said to let babies know that their parents are still there for them. However, these snippets of comfort are unlikely to have a lasting reassuring effect. The limited comfort recommended by some sleep training programs is rarely enough to help a baby settle down and peacefully drift off to sleep. While adults may consider a brief affectionate touch comforting and soothing, it is anything but from babies' point of view: all they know is that their parents are not doing what they need to relieve their distress and that most of the time Mom and Dad are *not* there to help them feel better.

As we saw in the previous chapter, babies need their parents to help them recover when they are upset because their brains are too immature to calm themselves down. Brief parental return visits and a little patting are rarely enough for babies to feel safe again and for the brain to transition from "on alert" to calm and relaxed. Babies often become very distressed when their parents walk out of the room shortly after coming in, as these parents' stories illustrate:

> When I went back in, I kept the settling to a minimum . . . me being in the room seemed to upset her. I guess she just thought she would be picked up and cuddled.

> We cannot go to Abby—the two times we went to her at bedtime, she cried twice as long as she usually does.

At four to six months of age, babies begin to develop *object permanence*—the ability to understand that something (or someone) exists even when we cannot see, feel, or hear it. However, it does not fully mature until a child is about two years old, and like so many aspects of infant development, it occurs at different rates in different children.[32] So, if babies cannot see, feel, or hear their mom or dad, as far as they are concerned, that parent has disappeared permanently.

This might be fine for a while if they are happily playing, but if they are alone and distressed, they cannot reassure themselves that their parents will return, which leaves them terrified and despairing. They have no way of knowing that their parents are just outside the bedroom door, listening to their screams. And even if babies *could* comprehend that Mom and Dad are right next to the door, it would be painful for them to know that they can hear them suffering but choose to do nothing about it.

Sleep Training: Being out of Attunement with Your Baby

In chapter 3, we examined how important feeling attuned to loving caregivers is for babies' brain development. We also learned how this feeling of attunement helps babies' brains forge the pathways that make it easier to cope well with stress. This gives us further insight into why sleep training is so risky. Babies left alone usually cry for their parents, meaning "come and help me feel all right again." When their parents don't return quickly or leave again before they feel calm and secure, babies' brains miss out on the much-needed experience of reattunement with their parents, and are left swimming in stress hormones.[33] This is called an "attachment rupture," and if it occurs repeatedly, it will negatively affect a baby's ability to recover from stressful situations later in life.

Sleep Training Is Tough on Parents

Parents often declare that sleep training is one of the hardest things they have ever done. This is not surprising because it directly undermines our deep biological compulsion to comfort our babies when they are distressed. Some parents said the following about sleep training:

Having to listen to your baby crying—it goes against every maternal instinct you have.

I was in floods of tears. How could I be so cruel to the most precious thing in the whole world?

My whole body was saying, "Go back in to her, give her the biggest hug possible, and tell her you'll nominate yourself for the worst-mother-of-the-year award tomorrow!"

I had to sit on [my husband] to keep him from rescuing her.

I found that vacuuming would help [distract me]; it drowned out the heartbreaking cries and made that dreaded five minutes at a time go past fairly fast!

It is literally gut-wrenching for me—listening to them cry is way worse than labor!

The crying was horrible. I sweated. I cried. My husband and I sat on the stairs with clock in hand, ready to time the intervals before going in to soothe her. We did this for four nights. On the third and fourth nights, our baby vomited. This was extremely traumatic for us.

These testaments show that sleep training is not a benign or gentle experience for anyone involved: if it is *heartbreaking, gut-wrenching,* and *traumatic* for an adult to *listen* to a baby's cries, it must be a devastating experience for the babies *doing* the crying.

Sleep training is stressful and emotionally painful for parents because they are biologically wired to respond to their babies' cries. Responding isn't simply a matter of choice, such as whether to go to a movie or concert on Friday night; magnetic resonance images (MRIs) of mothers' brains show that the hypothalamus and cingula are activated when their babies cry.[34] The result is that most mothers feel physically compelled to pick up and soothe their crying babies. Infant care and lactation consultant Anne Kohn explains it this way: "The impact of crying on a mother's nervous system is like sticking a fork in a power point [outlet]. Nature has designed parents to respond in that way so you will pick up your baby, not leave him to scream. If a baby is left to cry, he will get distressed and take twice as long to settle."[35]

Similarly, picking up our babies and cuddling them also affects parents' brains, giving us feelings of pleasure as a cascade of hormones, including dopamine, are released.[36] Unfortunately, advice to leave babies to cry themselves to sleep is so common in our culture that many parents who feel instinctively compelled to nurture their babies at bedtime start to lose confidence. They begin to think that there is something wrong with their parenting abilities, especially if health professionals tell them that this approach will be harmful; or, even worse, that they are to blame for their babies' sleep behavior. This misinformation stops many parents from simply enjoying their babies as they scramble to rectify a problem they didn't realize they had. Two moms said the following:

> I didn't know of any other options and felt ignorant as a first-time mom, so I assumed this was the "proper" way to get my child to sleep. So I "let them" instruct me on how to settle my three-week-old baby (just three weeks old!) with controlled crying. I felt totally disempowered, lost my confidence, and felt very disconnected from my baby for a long time, almost like she wasn't my daughter. Overall, my mental health was what suffered most, almost sending me to the ugly world of postnatal [postpartum] depression.

> I remember lying on the couch listening to her cry and cry, thinking motherhood wasn't supposed to be like this—and seriously considering not having more children. Yet I was convinced this was the only way to have a baby that was not in control of me and my marriage.

Pinky McKay, a parenting author and lactation consultant who works closely with parents, has this to say:

> I feel so sad at how normalized variations of controlled crying and rigid advice to schedule babies has become. I see parents

looking at their watches instead of their babies' cues; parents who are anxious about creating bad habits by cuddling their babies "too much" or comforting them to sleep; parents who spend so much time trying to make their babies sleep that they aren't getting to really enjoy that unique little person.[37]

Society's strong emphasis on teaching children to sleep independently can make some parents who take a more nurturing approach feel isolated, choosing to remain silent about their parenting style for fear of disapproval. One mother told us, "I don't tell people that I settle her with cuddles and rocking and patting, because I'm worried about their judgments."

Another disturbing effect of sleep training is how it can diminish parents' capacity to feel empathy for their children. Sleep training requires that parents deny or downplay their babies' suffering. They may be told, for instance, that their crying children are simply learning how to go to sleep alone,[38] find it difficult to understand what is happening,[39] or are angry and "shouting" for them to return.[40] Parents are even given practical advice on how to tune out their babies' cries. One parent was told the following by a health professional:

When you first leave your baby, it's not *too* bad so don't do anything. After the second visit, go and make coffee, which takes about five minutes. After the third visit, you have ten minutes to drink it. After the fourth visit, crack open a bottle of wine— it helps take your mind off your screaming baby, well, at least a little bit.

Other parents are advised to shut out their babies' cries by listening to music through headphones,[41] going to the other end of the house or outside,[42] or wearing earplugs.[43] At the heart of this advice is the denial of babies' emotional pain, which may dampen parents' empathy for their children over time. As one parent commented, "Once you have done this technique for a week, you will probably not find your baby's crying nearly as distressing."

Can Sleep Training Cause Babies to Emotionally Withdraw?

In chapter 2, we discussed how babies' healthy emotional development relies on responsive and sensitive care. If babies don't receive this kind of care, they may learn that they cannot trust their parents to offer comfort and reassurance when they feel sad or afraid, and that instead they must rely on themselves to manage difficult feelings.

When babies need their parents' attention, they let them know; for example, they will frown, then fuss, then cry, and then scream. The best outcome for babies is that their parents quickly notice their efforts for attention and do what they can to help them feel right again. When parents won't help their babies feel better, they feel sad, frustrated, and alarmed.

When infants are left alone in their cribs while feeling comfortable and secure, they may peacefully drift off to sleep. Yet in many instances, they need their parents' presence to feel safe and will cry and scream to communicate this. If this strategy does not bring back Mom and Dad, the crying will eventually diminish as most babies start to give up. In time, the infants or toddlers will seem to no longer need their parents at bedtime. Babies can cope if their parents fail to respond now and then; if this happens repeatedly, however, they can begin to feel helpless and will stop openly "telling" their parents when they need comfort and reassurance.[44] Instead, they focus their energies on dealing with the sadness and pain they feel at being ignored; in other words, they emotionally withdraw.[45] This is the way sleep training appears to work.

Psychologists describe the stages babies go through when they can't get needed help as first protest, then despair, and then detachment. Babies seem to experience these exact phases during sleep training.

Protest

Most parents who try sleep training are familiar with the protest stage during which babies become extremely fearful, distressed, and angry at being left alone. Children still hope that their parents will return, so they actively try to get them to come back.[46] The following two stories from parents illustrate this stage:

> We did the usual bedtime routine: I turned on her music and lights and then left the room. She screamed. She screamed some more. She cried. She banged her head against the cot [crib] in anger and frustration. She threw her milk on the floor, and she sounded almost hysterical. But it was in anger.

> She was shaking. Her face glistened in the light that streamed in from the door I had opened. Choking and sobbing, she threw her head against my chest and wailed. She was mad at me, and she was letting me know.

Many people dismiss babies' crying if they think it comes from anger. But anger is a powerful, intense emotion of self-protection: It is a common response to feeling hurt, threatened, or scared, and it can escalate to rage when people feel extremely threatened.[47] It helps children cry as hard as they can to try to get their parents to return.

Despair

Because babies cannot calm themselves when they feel distressed, they cry and scream—but they can't keep screaming forever. When their cries are unheeded, at some point they must start to conserve energy. Their brains begin to become overwhelmed with stress hormones, they begin to tire from trying to attract their parents' attention, and so they start to shut down.[48] Neurologically and emotionally, this is a very different process from that of babies who are soothed from distress to calm.

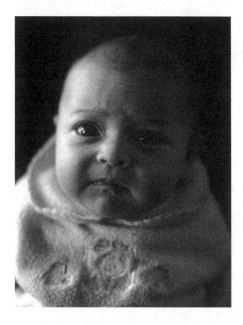

We can see that most babies who are left to cry will eventually become less angry but feel more despair about being left alone.[49] They feel increasingly hopeless about the chances of their parents returning. So the crying diminishes, and they sob and whimper rather than scream. Their cries don't sound so angry and intense. This is the point at which babies are starting to give up on their parents. Moms and dads have observed the following responses:

She's been stopping and starting; it's not hard wailing, just "Mommy, I'm alone. I don't like being alone." Crying.

The cry was completely different—more of a resigned cry rather than the frantic screaming of the night before.

It took one hour and twenty-five minutes, and even then he was whimpering as he slept.

Twenty minutes later—she's sort of doing this resigned, heaving sobbing now.

Parents are often told by professionals that the change in their babies' cries is a sign that sleep training is working. In fact, though, we should view it as a sign of babies feeling resigned and helpless.

Detachment

Finally, babies begin to withdraw and give up their efforts to get their parents' attention. At this stage, they appear fine and may fall asleep with no crying. But during the detachment phase, babies learn to suppress, rather than express, their feelings of sadness and despair. The following are stories from two mothers:

> Now, of course, she doesn't cry at all. We have had to duplicate the process a few times, as her schedule has been disrupted by teething, illness, or other stresses, but we have not had to be firm for longer than two nights. Now, she practically can't wait to get rid of me!

> She banged on our door for a half hour crying "Mommy, Daddy!" We called to her to go to bed, but to no avail, and eventually we heard her say to herself, "Mommy's at work," which almost broke my heart. But still, it didn't last many nights, and after that the threat of locking our door was usually enough to keep her in bed.

As child psychotherapist Margot Sunderland says, "A baby who is trained out of his instinct to cry on being separated from a parent should never be mistaken for being in a state of calm. His stress levels will have gone up, not down."[50]

Risks of the Protest, Despair, Detachment Process

Forcing a child to go through this process of protest, despair, and detachment creates particular risks. Babies who give up crying after long periods of distress in solitude have undergone very different neurological processes than those whose crying is soothed by comfort and reassurance. First, as we have seen, the stress levels of uncomforted babies have escalated. Second, the babies have cut themselves off from the world and from their own selves; they have detached from their feelings of distress and abandonment. This is known as *dissociation*.

For babies, dissociation is the last coping strategy available when their other attempts to alleviate distress are exhausted. It happens when their brains transition from hyperaroused fear to a state of hopelessness and helplessness; when they have no option but to shut themselves off. It is akin to what animals do when they feign death in response to a life-threatening situation.[51]

If stress-induced dissociation occurs repeatedly in infancy, shutting down can become embedded in the brain as a way of dealing with high-stress situations. This means that when faced with stressful events in the future, such as job interviews or intense conflicts with a partner, people may dissociate. The tendency to shut down and detach is extremely detrimental because it makes it difficult, or even impossible, to deal with situations rationally and effectively. We asked Allan N. Schore, one of the world's leading infant neuroscientists, for his opinion on sleep training, and he offered this insight: "Infants who habitually dissociate in the transition from wake to sleep states would experience altered brain chemistry during critical periods when the sleep mechanism is forming. These infants would stop crying, which might be behaviorally interpreted as a normal event, but indeed this would be anything but normal."[52]

The protest, despair, detachment process illustrates how sleep training works: By teaching babies to expect that their parents will *not* come to offer comfort when called. Yet babies develop optimally when they feel secure, loved, and that they *can* rely on their parents to provide comfort when they need it.

What Are Possible Long-Term Consequences of Sleep Training?

In the short term, sleep training clearly causes babies to feel insecure. We hear so many stories of infants becoming clingy and extrasensitive during the sleep training process. For example, one mother said, "Prior to [controlled crying] he was a happy little independent baby, who would laugh all day, go to anyone, and happily play by himself for hours. Now he is very clingy and sobby during the day, won't go to others, won't even sit on his own, and screams when I leave the room."

As we noted earlier in this chapter, whether sleep training causes lasting emotional insecurity has not been determined: To date, no credible research has examined the connection between sleep training and emotional security. However, we do have a wealth of research on the criteria for healthy emotional development and the effects of nonresponsiveness to babies' cries, which sheds light on the potentially harmful effects of this practice. Repeatedly leaving babies to cry alone can precipitate negative long-term consequences.[53]

Infant Amnesia—Do Babies' Experiences Have an Impact Later in Life?

You may have heard people say that babies won't be harmed by being left to cry because they won't remember the experience. While it's true that people cannot recall what happens to them when they are babies (remembering actual occurrences is called *explicit memory*), the experiences of babies and toddlers are stored in another type of memory called *implicit memory*.[54] Deeply stressful and traumatic events are recorded in the brain's amygdala.[55]

If people are unconsciously reminded of trauma or extreme stress they experienced in infancy, they can react to the memory without being consciously aware of having had a memory.[56] For example, children who felt deeply abandoned during sleep training in infancy may become intensely distressed in situations in which they sense the possibility of being abandoned again—by their parents, peers, or in later years, romantic partners. This seemingly irrational behavior is actually in reaction to memories of which they have no conscious recall.

The brains of babies who are repeatedly left in highly stressed states are permanently changed.[57] When infants become frantically distressed, their brains are flooded with stress hormones and move to code red alert, a state referred to as *hypermetabolic* or—literally—

"burning up."[58] This neurotoxic state can cause damage to the emotional centers of babies' brains: Cells can shrink and die, and some of those new connections that they have been busily building (as discussed in chapter 3) can be eliminated. Babies in high survival mode also have little energy for the brain growth they need.

Because emotional security develops when children are consistently and sensitively soothed when upset, repeatedly allowing them to experience preventable distress, even at sleep time, can potentially prevent the establishment of a secure bond between parent and child. As we have seen, sleep training can be traumatic for some babies and could detrimentally affect their ability to cope with stress throughout life. Trauma can have a devastating impact on a child's development and psychological health; consequences include excessive crying and inability to be soothed, intense distress during transitions, intractable tantrums, somatic complaints, poor frustration tolerance, aggression, noncompliance, accident-prone behavior, and excessive separation anxiety.[59] Parents may not realize their babies have been traumatized because these traits also fall within the more severe realm of normal infant and toddler behavior; therefore, they may not link them with sleep training, believing their children are just being difficult or naughty.

There are also a great many unknowns about the neurological and emotional impact of sleep training: Could it increase the risks of later problems such as sleep onset difficulties, anxiety at nighttime, or insomnia? Furthermore, could it lead to more complex emotional problems? Dr. Daniel Hughes, a childhood trauma specialist, believes so:

> Since crying for infants and preverbal children is the primary way that they express their attachment behaviors, to ignore their cries most likely will create problems with the development of attachment security. Certainly I am not suggesting that periodic inability to respond or delay in responding to crying will be detrimental to an infant or young child. My concern involves the efforts to train a child not to cry when in mild

to moderate distress, to not communicate with a parent when in a negative emotional state. If successful, parents may discover that their child stops seeking their attention, comfort, and guidance around a range of issues as he or she develops. The child may develop a habit of "going it alone" in ways that parents will deeply regret in years to come. Whatever sleep improvement the parents may receive when the child is young may well be lost when the parents spend sleepless nights when their child enters adolescence and decides not to rely on his or her parents.[60]

Hughes explains how it is well worth investing your time and energy *now* to respond to your child's cries and foster attachment security. Going for the "quick fix" in your baby's early life may have great costs in later years.

The Good News

Parents who have practiced sleep training may feel guilty when they learn about its possible impact on a baby's development—even though they did what they believed to be best at the time. The good news is that with patience and persistence, it is possible to amend many of sleep training's negative effects.

The brain is capable of making new connections throughout life, but it takes longer to do so in later childhood and adulthood than in infancy. This means that many of the effects of difficult early childhood experiences can be healed by sensitive parental care; children can come to trust their parents again, and new emotional bonds can be forged. The healing process can take time, though, and may require a lot of patience.

If you are concerned that sleep training has had a detrimental impact on your child, there are some excellent books that explore how to emotionally connect with your child (see "Suggested Reading" on pages 197 to 200). You can also take some practical steps. If your children seem to be frightened of their cribs or beds after sleep training, think about how you can modify the sleep environment so it doesn't remind them of that painful experience. For example, could you change the bedding and move the position of the crib, or is baby old enough to start sleeping in a bed? You could also gradually build new and positive associations by helping your children feel safe in their bedrooms—maybe by holding, rocking, massaging, and singing to them there. Another option is to move baby into your bed to experience nighttime closeness (see pages 115 to 116 for information about safe bed sharing).

The most important thing you can do to lessen the impact of any serious distress is to forgive yourself if you feel a child has been hurt by your actions; remember that you did your best with the information you had available at the time. Self-forgiveness will allow you to focus on your children and respond sensitively to their needs, speeding them along the road to recovery.

This chapter discussed the main elements of sleep training programs and their possible negative consequences for a child's development. Despite its popularity, sleep training is clearly tough on babies and their parents. It nearly always causes distress, sometimes intense and prolonged. But sleep training is not the only option available to parents—in the next part of the book, we turn to how parents can respond to their baby's sleep issues in gentle, sensitive ways.

Key Points

- The essential ingredient of sleep training is withholding parental love and comfort—this emotional deprivation is deeply upsetting for babies on an intrinsic level.

- Although certain forms of sleep training may sound benign, all methods usually cause considerable distress for babies and parents.

- The changes to a baby's sleep brought about by sleep training are often impermanent. Consequently, many children have to endure repeated episodes of sleep training.

- Parents can assist in the maturation of babies' sleep by responding gently to their biological and emotional needs—not by leaving babies to cry, scream, or even vomit.

NOTES

1. Mahatma Gandhi and Krishna Kripalani, *All Men Are Brothers: Autobiographical Reflections* (New York: Continuum International Publishing, 2004), 72.

2. David Kaiser, "Love and Dependence: Harry Harlow Revisited," *What's New in Neurofeedback* 8, no. 12 (December 2005), http://start.eegspectrum.com/Newsletter/dec2005.htm (accessed October 2006).

3. John B. Watson, *Psychological Care of Infant and Child* (New York: W. W. Norton & Company, 1928), 87; and Robert Karen, *Becoming Attached: First Relationships and How They Shape Our Capacity to Love* (New York: Oxford University Press, 1994), 4–5.

4. Tizzie Hall, "Night Cries," *Practical Parenting* (December 2003): 57.

5. Brian Symon, *Silent Nights: Overcoming Sleep Problems in Babies and Children* (South Melbourne, Australia: Oxford University Press, 1998), 67.

6. Charles E. Schaefer and Michael R. Petronko, *Teach Your Baby to Sleep through the Night* (London: Thorsons, 1993), 47.

7. Richard Ferber, *Solve Your Child's Sleep Problems* (St. Leonards, Australia: Dorling Kindersley, 1999), 67.

8. Christopher Green, *Babies! A Parents' Guide to Enjoying Baby's First Year*, 2nd ed. (East Roseville, Australia: Simon & Schuster Australia, 2001), 178–179.

9. Rosey Cummings, Karen Houghton, and Ann Williams, *Sleep Right, Sleep Tight: A Practical, Proven Guide to Solving Your Baby's Sleep Problems* (Sydney: Doubleday, 2000), 66, 67; and Maree Viotto, *It's Time to Sleep: How to Get Your Child Sleeping Like a Baby* (book and DVD) (Melbourne, Australia: Hybrid, 2004).

10. Tizzie Hall, "Sleep Routines for Newborns," *Practical Parenting* (July 2005): 80–83; and Symon, *Silent Nights*, 93.

11. Symon, *Silent Nights*, 108; Cummings, Houghton, and Williams, *Sleep Right, Sleep Tight*, 112; and Ferber, *Solve Your Child's Sleep Problems*.

12. Kaz Cooke, *Kid-Wrangling: The Real Guide to Caring for Babies, Toddlers and Preschoolers* (Melbourne, Australia: Viking, 2003), 278.

13. Marc Weissbluth, *Healthy Sleep Habits, Happy Child: A Step-by-Step Programme for a Good Night's Sleep* (London: Vermilion, 2005), 132.

14. Robin Barker, "Teaching-to-Sleep Guide," *Totline: The Playgroup NSW Journal* 4 (2005): 10–11.

15. Daniel J. Siegel and Mary Hartzell, *Parenting from the Inside Out: How a Deeper Self-Understanding Can Help You Raise Children Who Thrive* (New York: Jeremy P. Tarcher/Penguin, 2003), 200.

16. Ibid.

17. Jodi A. Mindell, "Empirically Supported Treatments in Pediatric Psychology: Bedtime Refusal and Night Wakings in Young Children," *Journal of Pediatric Psychology* 24, no. 6 (1999): 465–481; and Paul Ramchandani, Luci Wiggs, Vicky Webb, and Gregory Stores, "A Systematic Review of Treatment of Settling Problems and Night Waking in Young Children," *British Medical Journal* 320 (January 22, 2000): 209–213.

18. Harriet Hiscock, Jordana Bayer, Lisa Gold, Anne Hampton, Obioha C. Ukoumunne, and Melissa Wake, "Improving Infant Sleep and Maternal Mental Health: A Cluster Randomised Trial," *Archives of Disease in Childhood* 92, no. 11 (2007): 952–958.

19. Berndt Eckerberg, "Treatment of Sleep Problems in Families with Young Children: Effects of Treatment on Family Well-Being," *Acta Paediatrica* 93, no. 1 (2004): 126–134.

20. Klaus Minde, André Faucon, and Suki Falkner, "Sleep Problems in Toddlers: Effects of Treatment on Their Daytime Behavior," *Journal of the American Academy of Child & Adolescent Psychiatry* 33, no. 8 (1994): 1114–1121; Karyn G. France, "Behaviour Characteristics and Security in Sleep-Disturbed Infants Treated with Extinction," *Journal of Pediatric Psychology* 17, no. 4 (1992): 467–475; Frederick W. Seymour, Gay Bayfield, Phyllis Brock, and Mary During, "Management of Night-Waking in Young Children," *Australian Journal of Family Therapy* 4, no. 4 (1983): 217–223; and note 19 above.

21. For a discussion of such tools, see Lisa J. Berlin, Yair Ziv, Lisa Amaya-

Jackson, and Mark T. Greenberg, eds., *Enhancing Early Attachments: Theory, Research, Intervention, and Policy* (New York: Guilford Press, 2005), 67.

22. Eckerberg, "Treatment of Sleep Problems in Families with Young Children," 132.

23. Siegel and Hartzell, *Parenting from the Inside Out*, 87, 185.

24. Bert Powell, "Baby Bonding Video," by Andrea Palpant and David Tanner (North by Northwest Productions, Circle of Security: Early Intervention Program for Parents and Children), www.circleofsecurity.org (accessed October 5, 2006).

25. Erik Hesse, "The Adult Attachment Interview: Historical and Current Perspectives," in *Handbook of Attachment: Theory, Research, and Clinical Applications*, eds. Jude Cassidy and Phillip R. Shaver (New York: Guilford Press, 1999), 395–433.

26. Alicia F. Lieberman, "The Emotional Life of the Toddler," *The Signal: Newsletter of the World Association for Infant Mental Health* 2, no. 4 (October–December 1994): 1–4.

27. New Jersey Disaster Mental Health, "What Is Trauma?" www.njdisastermentalhealth.org/wh_tr00.htm (accessed March 2006).

28. Centre for Community Child Health, Royal Children's Hospital, Melbourne, "Controlled Comforting: A Quick Reference Guide," http://raisingchildren.net.au/articles/controlled_comforting.html (accessed October 2006).

29. Jean Kunhardt, "Sleep Training," http://newyork.urbanbaby.com/community/expert/021200.html (accessed October 2006).

30. Isla Lonie, "Long-Term Effects of Controlled Crying," personal communication (email), April 9, 2006.

31. References quoted by Isla Lonie (above): Allan N. Schore, *Affect Regulation and the Origin of the Self: The Neurobiology of Emotional Development* (Hillsdale, New Jersey: Lawrence Erlbaum Associates, 1994); Allan N. Schore, "The Experience-Dependent Maturation of a Regulatory System in the Orbital Prefrontal Cortex and the Origin of Developmental Psychopathology," *Development and Psychopathology* 8 (1996): 59–87; Allan N. Schore, "Early Organization of the Nonlinear Right Brain and Development of a Predisposition to Psychiatric Disorders," *Development and Psychopathology* 9 (1997): 595–632; and Colwyn Trevarthen and Kenneth J. Aitken, "Brain

Development, Infant Communication, and Empathy Disorders: Intrinsic Factors in Child Mental Health," *Development and Psychopathology* 6 (1994): 597–633.

32. M. Keith Moore and Andrew N. Meltzoff, "New Findings on Object Permanence: A Developmental Difference between Two Types of Occlusion," *British Journal of Developmental Psychology* 17 (1999): 563–584.

33. Allan N. Schore, *Affect Dysregulation and Disorders of the Self* (New York: W. W. Norton & Company, 2003), 114–115.

34. Jeffrey P. Lorberbaum, John D. Newman, Judy R. Dubno, Amy R. Horwitz, Ziad Nahas, et al., "Feasibility of Using MRI to Study Mothers Responding to Infant Cries," *Depression and Anxiety* 10, no. 3 (1999): 99–104.

35. Anne Kohn, interview, March 26, 2006.

36. Margot Sunderland, *The Science of Parenting: Practical Guidance on Sleep, Crying, Play and Building Emotional Wellbeing for Life* (London: Dorling Kindersley, 2006), 191.

37. Pinky McKay, personal communication (email), February 20, 2006.

38. Ferber, *Solve Your Child's Sleep Problems*.

39. Cummings, Houghton, and Williams, *Sleep Right, Sleep Tight*, 19.

40. Hall, "Night Cries," 56–57.

41. Cummings, Houghton, and Williams, *Sleep Right, Sleep Tight*, 29.

42. Catherine Fowler and Patricia Gornall, *How to Stay Sane in Your Baby's First Year: The Tresillian Guide*, 3rd ed. (East Roseville, Australia: Simon & Schuster Australia, 2001), 122.

43. Weissbluth, *Healthy Sleep Habits, Happy Child*.

44. Edward Z. Tronick and Andrew F. Gianino, "Interactive Mismatch and Repair: Challenges to the Coping Infant," *Zero to Three: Bulletin of the National Center for Clinical Infant Programs* 6, no. 3 (1986): 1–6; and Australian Association for Infant Mental Health, *Position Paper 2: Responding to Babies' Cues* (September 2006), www.aaimhi.org/documents/position%20papers/Position%20Paper%202.pdf (accessed December 2008).

45. Tronick and Gianino, "Interactive Mismatch and Repair," 1–6; and Lynne Murray and Colwyn Trevarthen, "Emotional Regulation of Interactions between Two-Month-Olds and Their Mothers," in *Social Perception in Infants*, eds. Tiffany M. Field and Nathan A. Fox (Norwood, New Jersey: Ablex

Publishing Corporation, 1985), 177–197.

46. Roger Kobak, "The Emotional Dynamics of Disruptions in Attachment Relationships: Implications for Theory, Research, and Clinical Intervention," in *Handbook of Attachment*, eds. Cassidy and Shaver, 21–43.

47. Babette Rothschild, *The Body Remembers: The Psychophysiology of Trauma and Trauma Treatment* (New York: W. W. Norton & Company, 2000), 61.

48. Daniel J. Siegel, *The Developing Mind: How Relationships and the Brain Interact to Shape Who We Are* (New York: Guilford Press, 1999).

49. See note 46 above.

50. Sunderland, *The Science of Parenting*, 79.

51. Rothschild, *The Body Remembers*, 49; and Allan N. Schore, "Attachment Trauma and the Developing Right Brain: Origins of Pathological Dissociation," in *Dissociation and the Dissociative Disorders: DSM-V and Beyond*, eds. Paul F. Dell and John A. O'Neil (New York: Routledge, 2009).

52. Allan N. Schore, personal communication (email), December 20, 2005.

53. Australian Association for Infant Mental Health, *Position Paper 2* (accessed December 2008).

54. Siegel and Hartzell, *Parenting from the Inside Out*, 23; and Rothschild, *The Body Remembers*, 37.

55. Siegel and Hartzell, *Parenting from the Inside Out*, 175; and Rothschild, *The Body Remembers*.

56. Siegel and Hartzell, *Parenting from the Inside Out*, 23; and Rothschild, *The Body Remembers*.

57. National Scientific Council on the Developing Child, "Excessive Stress Disrupts the Architecture of the Developing Brain," www.developing child.net/pubs/wp-abstracts/wp3.html (accessed March 2006).

58. Schore, "Attachment Trauma and the Developing Right Brain."

59. Alicia F. Lieberman, "Traumatic Stress and Quality of Attachment: Reality and Internalization in Disorders of Infant Mental Health," *Infant Mental Health Journal* 25, no. 4 (2004): 336–351.

60. Daniel Hughes, personal communication (email), February 23, 2006.

PART 2: PRACTICE

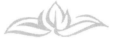

Gentle Ways to Help Your Baby (and You)

CHAPTER 5

Gentle Approaches to Help Your Baby Sleep

~⁂~

*We need . . . to adopt the emotional tone and caregiving attitudes
that are most helpful in meeting each child's unique needs.
Parents should be wary of any "one-size-fits-all" approach
that oversimplifies something as complex as child rearing.*[1]
STANLEY GREENSPAN

Helping babies go to sleep can be difficult. In fact, it is one of the main
reasons parents turn to sleep training. In this chapter, we give advice
on how you can gently help your baby sleep—starting with a baby-
friendly sleep routine. Then we look at settling techniques for different ages and what to do when you're ready to change techniques—
when your current tried-and-true "go to sleep" method stops working,
for example.

Unlike other authors, we do not offer a one-size-fits-all sleep solution. All babies' sleep needs are different, and they evolve over time.
We don't promise that your baby will necessarily sleep through the
night (in fact, despite some grand claims for sleep training, even its
supporters acknowledge a 30 percent "failure rate").[2] However, we
do guarantee that these techniques have worked well for other parents, and all the methods are respectful of the developmental needs
of babies and toddlers. We include the ideas of two very experienced

nurses, Marianne Nicholson and Anne Kohn, who have worked with hundreds of parents and babies.[3] In the next chapter, we discuss common sleep problems and how to cope with them.

Develop a Baby-Friendly Sleep Routine

A big surprise for many new parents is that babies, unlike puppies and kittens, do not always just go to sleep by themselves. We saw how baby sleep is very different from adult sleep in chapter 1. In practice, this means that babies need help to go to sleep, both at nighttime and at nap time. But, as we will explain, you can ease off the amount of assistance you give over time. "Gentle Techniques for Specific Age Groups" (pages 120–123) provides a list of effective settling techniques for babies of various ages.

Routines can really help set up a nice sleepy environment, but there are vastly different types of routines. Some baby books offer rigid schedules that promise to create contented babies who sleep through the night early and easily.[4] These books map out exactly what time to feed babies, when to play with them, when they should sleep, and when they should vomit on your last clean shirt (okay, we made that last one up!).[5] Occasionally and by chance, some babies' natural rhythms do fit well with these tight guidelines, but most families find that trying to wedge their cuddly round babies into sharp square holes just makes everybody miserable. As one mother said, "I've seen my friends get their babies into these routines, but it takes an awful lot of crying." Another mother shared the following:

> Now that I look back, I think that by trying to change her behavior, trying to impose a routine, we probably created the problem—we took an easy baby and made it hard work. I feel angry and sad [about it] now. I would have enjoyed my daugh-

ter's babyhood so much more if I had had the courage to follow my own instincts. All the needless time and anxiety trying to fix something that wasn't broken—I really regret that.

Naturally, we are not aiming for a lot of crying, and we don't want to control every moment of your day—we want to help you create routines that relax babies and give them cues that it's time for bed. A typical nighttime routine might involve bath, massage, pajamas, breast-feed or bottle, books, a hug and a kiss, and off to sleep. A daytime routine might include singing and music. Some babies are soothed by a CD of special lullabies or songs you sing at every sleep time. Nonverbal signs can also cue babies for sleep. In the first twelve months of Beth's youngest son's life, Matthew knew that being swaddled was the signal for sleep (firmly when he was a newborn and then more loosely as he grew). After about twelve months—when he was no longer interested in being swaddled—Beth created a "sign" that meant it was time for sleep: she would put the palms of her hands together and lay her head on her hands. When she combined this sign with saying, "Time for sleepy bye-byes," it meant that it was time for bed. Before long, Matthew began pressing the chubby palms of his hands against his head when he heard "Time for sleepy bye-byes."

Routines work because the repetition of particular soothing sounds and behaviors (called *sleep associations*) helps babies know what is coming next—sleep! In this way, routines trigger the relaxation and sleep response. Anni's son Karl (now nine years old) still asks for his baby bedtime song, "Jumping Sheep," if he has a hard day.

The key to effective sleep routines is keeping them simple and consistent: simple, because you want the other parent or caregivers to be able to follow your routine; and consistent, because repetition builds the expectation that it's bedtime and encourages sleepiness. If your bedtime routine isn't working, or stops working, changing it a little can help, as this mother found:

I knew a bedtime routine was important and gave my son a bath before bed, but as soon as I lay down with him to read him a book, he wanted to have a breast-feed, because this was where I usually fed him to sleep. Hence our "bedtime routine" was very short and not very effective! It was such a simple suggestion, but when a nurse suggested that I put a chair in his room and read to him from the chair, we were able to have several books before bed, and it really helped him settle down.

How Feeding Relates to Sleep

Feeding and baby sleep are closely related. Babies often fall asleep while feeding, and, of course, they wake up to feed. Parents receive stern advice about never feeding their baby to sleep, yet clear thinking and examining the evidence about feeding and sleeping issues can help parents gain a new perspective.

One question a lot of mothers ask us is whether they should breast-feed their babies to sleep. Sometimes they have heard that if babies get used to falling asleep this way, it will prevent them from learning to sleep independently and from getting a good night's sleep. Yet, despite dire warnings, many babies relax on the breast and love to drift off in their mother's arms—and mothers love this too. All babies who are breast-fed to sleep eventually learn to go to sleep without the breast. One mother explained as follows:

> From about four months to now [seven months], she has been breast-fed to sleep—it always works, she's happy, it doesn't take long, and it's healthy for her too. For a while, I held some guilt about breast-feeding her to sleep; however, it just felt so natural that deep down I knew it was the right thing to do.

Whether or not you breast-feed your baby to sleep (and for how long) is something you and your baby must work out together.

Nourishing Your Baby:
Why Breast-Feeding Is So Important

Breast milk is unequalled in promoting the health of babies—not only while they are nursing but also for the rest of their lives.[6] According to the American Academy of Pediatrics, breast-feeding reduces babies' risk of developing many diseases, including bacterial meningitis, diarrhea, respiratory tract infection, necrotizing enterocolitis (serious infection of the intestine), otitis media (middle ear infection), and urinary tract infection. Other studies have shown decreased rates of diabetes, lymphomas, leukemia, Hodgkin's disease, asthma, obesity, and gastroenteritis in breast-fed children.

Economists estimate that billions of dollars in annual health-care costs for sick infants would be saved if breast-feeding rates and duration were increased.[7] The protection offered by breast-feeding grows with the amount a baby receives, so the less often you replace breast milk with formula, the less often your baby is likely to become ill.[8]

Health professionals do a great disservice to families when they tell parents that breast-feeding is best but that formula feeding is a very close substitute. With the right information and support, almost all mothers are capable of breast-feeding their infants;[9] however, they will be far less motivated to do so (and less likely to receive essential support from partners, family, friends, and their community) if factual information about the importance of breast-feeding is not readily available. While we understand that an unsuccessful experience with breast-feeding is a matter of great regret for many mothers, this is no reason to underplay the significance of breast milk to infants' health.

Besides breast-feeding, other feeding issues can occur during sleep time. "Fill up their tummies, and they will sleep better" is quite common advice for new parents. At about four to five months of age, as babies become more alert and engaged with the world, many begin to wake frequently. Mistaking this as a sign of hunger, some parents assume that this night waking means babies are ready for solids or that feeding them some formula will help. However, there are exceptionally good reasons not to introduce solids before six months or to give formula to breast-fed babies in an effort to make them less wakeful. There is no research to show that the early introduction of solids makes babies wake less often. Also, babies cannot benefit from solids until they are developmentally ready.[10] According to the Australian National Health and Medical Research Council, babies' kidneys and immature digestive systems are not ready for solid food until six months of age.[11] Introducing solids early exposes infants to the risk of food allergies and obesity.

Introducing formula to breast-fed babies in the hope of making them sleep can have unintended consequences. Even just one bottle of formula changes the acidity levels in babies' bowels and increases the chance of bowel infection and diarrhea.[12] It may then take up to a month of exclusive breast-feeding for the digestive flora in a baby's system to return to normal. Furthermore, introducing formula can also decrease the length of time that babies breast-feed and can even spell the end of breast-feeding altogether. Because milk is easier to

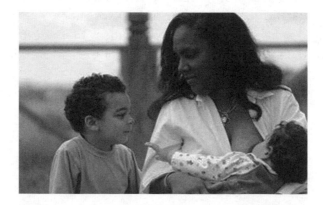

get out of a bottle than the breast, many infants refuse the breast soon after bottles are introduced. Also, when babies drink formula, they are removing less milk from their mothers' breasts and so reduce their mothers' production of milk.

Make Sure Your Baby Is Tired

Older babies and toddlers need to be clearly tired before you start any settling techniques, or they won't go to sleep, and you'll end up feeling frustrated. It's important to make sure babies are physically tired at bedtime. This means making time for lots of physical activity every day—in the park, the yard, or even an obstacle course through the house. You've no doubt heard that babies show "tired signs," such as jerky body movements, eye rubbing, back arching, and becoming fussy. If you pay close attention to your baby, you'll soon start to notice her tired signs. During the daytime, these signs are a cue to stop playtime and start preparing her for sleep—by having some quiet time, then rocking or patting or placing her in the crib—whatever works for you and your baby.

Being in sync with your baby's signals and tiredness cycle can really help save time and energy, as this mother observed:

> It's important you catch these [tired] signs and put the baby to bed, as an overtired baby is one that finds it hard to sleep. . . . At eighteen months, Tasman still has very obvious tired signs—he rubs his eyes and, if I miss that cue, he gets a little bit hyperactive. If I miss that window of opportunity for sleep, it can mean a lot of books need to be read to him.

To avoid these types of problems, figure out approximately what time your baby begins to get tired, and start your bedtime routine a half an hour before that.

Settle Yourself to Help Settle Your Baby

If *you* are unsettled, it can be difficult to help your baby settle. Child psychotherapist and author Margot Sunderland explains that "your tone is everything, and if you are tense, uptight, irritated, or angry your [baby can] feel too unsafe to go to sleep."[13] Infant care and lactation consultant Anne Kohn puts it this way: "If you're in top gear, you can't get your baby into neutral." Former child and family nurse practitioner Marianne Nicholson agrees, noting the following:

> Babies are very good at noticing when something's up; for example, if Mom's thinking "Look, I've got six emails that I've got to send, and I just want you to go to sleep now so I can tick these things off my list," baby says, "Aha! She's wound up about something. I'd better stay awake and see what's happening." So if Mom can get someone to walk her baby around the block while she sends her emails, then she relaxes and baby says, "There's nothing worrying Mom, I can go to sleep!"

Now, we realize that what we are suggesting can feel almost impossible at times. It can be horribly frustrating when your baby is awake but should be asleep, in your opinion! The more agitated you are, however, the less you will be able to help your baby sleep, so it is imperative that you manage your feelings. Try the following tips to calm yourself down while you settle your baby:

- Play soothing music.

- Practice deep breathing.

- Try your best to accept any situation. Remember that your baby will sleep eventually, and although it may feel like the world will collapse if your baby doesn't sleep right away, it won't.

- Notice what's happening in your body: Which parts feel good? Which parts feel tense? If your muscles feel especially stiff or cramped, try relaxing them with a heating pad.

- Do your best to let go of other concerns, perhaps even telling yourself aloud, "I can wait until tomorrow to make that phone call if I can't do it today" or "I can't force my baby to sleep."
- Try to remember how much you love your baby: how soft her skin is and how nice she smells.

Rachel, a mother of four, sums it up well:

I have always found that if I wanted to have the babies asleep by a certain time, I could be guaranteed they wouldn't be! This was usually because I was expecting someone, wanted to get something done, or needed to go out without them. I would get very angry and feel stressed if the babies wouldn't sleep. It took me a long time to accept that perhaps they didn't want to sleep. Once I acknowledged that, I could get on with things, even if the baby wasn't asleep.

Co-Sleeping

Although it's not for everyone, co-sleeping is an option that works for many families. Some parents find that having their babies sleep with them in bed, in a crib in their room, or next to their bed with the crib side off or down is the best way for everyone to get a good night's sleep:[14]

Bringing our babies into bed has minimized sleep loss and kept us going for nearly ten years!

Although getting to sleep at nighttime has sometimes been a challenge for us, night-waking has never really been a drama as we have a family bed. Tasman stirs from two to ten times a night to breast-feed but neither he nor I really notice: he doesn't actually wake up and I don't always.

These stories show that co-sleeping allows babies to feed often without disturbing their mothers too much, giving everyone a (relatively) undisturbed night's sleep. We discuss how to sleep safely with your baby in the following section.

Create a Safe Sleeping Environment

Wherever babies sleep, they should sleep safely to minimize the risk of SIDS (sudden infant death syndrome) and sleeping accidents. Abide by these general safety guidelines no matter where your baby sleeps (specific guidelines for bed sharing and crib sleeping follow):[15]

- Lay babies on their backs—not on the side or stomach.

- Have a clean, firm mattress. Make sure the mattress protector fits tightly so the baby's bed feels firm.

- Use light cotton or wool blankets—no duvets or synthetic fabrics. You may avoid the use of blankets and covers altogether by dressing babies in sleepers (one-piece coverall pajamas) or by putting them in specially designed sleeping bags.

- Keep baby chemical-free—use soap and water to clean crib mattresses (rather than chemical cleaners) and do not dry-clean bedding.

- Use a washable mattress cover.

- Regularly air out the mattress.

- Keep babies' sleep environments free of cords—such as from toys, cell phones, electronics, or blinds.

- Keep babies' environments smoke-free, and do not let anyone smoke near your babies.

- Make sure that pets cannot enter the room where babies are sleeping.

- Do not overheat babies (as a general guide, they need the same number of layers as you do).

- Do not use electric blankets, hot water bottles, or heating pads because overheating increases the chance of SIDS.

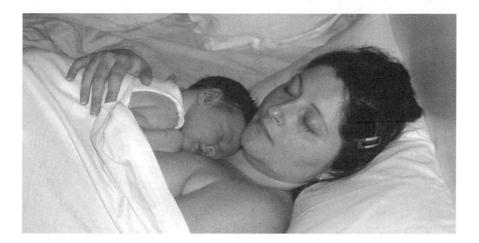

Safe Bed Sharing

- Do not sleep with babies on waterbeds, soft mattresses, or on sofas or sofa beds—babies need to sleep on firm surfaces.
- Make sure babies' faces cannot be covered by anything such as pillows, stuffed animals, long hair, and so on.
- Make sure babies cannot fall out of bed or get stuck between the mattress and the adjoining wall or furniture.
- Do not swaddle babies too tightly—this can restrict movement and may make them too hot.
- Do not let babies sleep with other children or pets.
- Avoid wearing nightwear that has string ties, long ribbons, and so on.

Do not bed share if any of the following describes either parent:

- Obese.
- A smoker (no matter what, where, or when you smoke).
- Intoxicated by alcohol, sedatives, or any other drugs that make you sleepy.

- Unusually tired (to a point where you would find it difficult to respond to your baby).

- Ill or has a condition that would make it difficult to respond to your baby.

Safe Crib Sleeping[16]

- Keep your baby's crib in your room for the first six months, as this has been found to significantly reduce the risk of SIDS.[17]

- Lay babies "feet to foot" (with baby's feet to the foot of the mattress) so they can't slip down under the blankets.

- Keep babies' faces and heads uncovered.

- Do not use crib bumpers for babies under one year old.

- Do not put soft toys, quilts, duvets, or pillows where babies sleep.

- Securely tuck in bedclothes so that bedding is not loose.

- Before you buy a crib (including portable cribs), check the label to make sure it meets design standards.

- A crib mattress should be the right size: make sure there is no more than a 1-inch (25mm) gap between the mattress, the crib sides, and the ends of the crib.

Help Your Baby Settle
Down and Fall Asleep

During the first few months, many infants naturally fall asleep while breast- or bottle-feeding. Some babies like being patted as they fall asleep, while others like being rocked in their parents' arms or in a rocking chair. Walking around with baby in a sling also works well for many fussy babies. With little babies, the important thing is not to put them down or stop patting or feeding too early. You may recall from chapter 1 that young babies enter sleep from the light sleep state, so if you stop settling them too quickly, they wake very easily and you have to start over. So wait until babies' movements and eye flickering calm down, or they suddenly feel "heavy" in your arms (usually after about twenty minutes)—this is the time to put them in the crib and slip away.

Some babies find it hard to relax enough to go to sleep. These fussy or high-need babies usually require extra help at bedtime or nap time; many wake very easily too. Parents of these babies need to be creative and patient with their settling techniques. If your baby does find it difficult to settle down and remain asleep, it is certainly worth examining the lists in the next chapter; an underlying physical or emotional problem might be the cause. However, some babies may just have "high needs" for comfort and can be easily overstimulated and overwhelmed.

The key to helping fussy babies sleep is to figure out what works best for them. Some sensitive infants seem to need a lot of movement to settle down. For instance, Anni found dancing to music with a steady beat usually helped her son Ben go to sleep. Reducing stimulation as much as possible at sleep time (for example, dim lighting, no sound, and gently rocking or patting) is also an effective settling technique for some of these babies. Others seem to find soft, gentle background noise very calming, such as soothing music, lullabies, or story tapes. However, we advise against using white noise, such as the sound of a vacuum cleaner, radio static, or recorded mechanical noises. While some parents have reported that these types of sounds seem to relax babies, recent research shows that excessive, indiscriminate noise can overstimulate young mammals' developing brains and should therefore be avoided.[18]

Getting fussy babies to fall asleep is one thing, but keeping them asleep can be a challenge, even if you put them down in apparent deep sleep. Parents of constant wakers have found that it sometimes works to keep a baby upright, moving, or both. If a baby has reflux, organizing an upright sleeping position frequently helps. Constant movement can be more difficult; Ben's dad used to put him into the fold of a huge sweater, hold each end, and rock him back and forth every time he stirred. Unfortunately, while effective, this technique was fairly exhausting. Other parents find the following types of movement to be helpful: rocking in a rocking chair, baby swing, or hammock (some are battery operated—giving babies the movement they need and the rest you need!), driving around in a car, and walking while baby sleeps in a sling or baby carriage (if you want to get some exercise too). Of course, whichever technique you decide to use with your sensitive little one, make sure it is safe (and won't hurt your back).

Is Eye Contact Okay at Sleep Time?

Moms and dads are often told to avoid eye contact with their baby at sleep time so he or she is not tempted to engage in play. This may be fine by babies if they are content and relaxed, but if they feel upset, eye contact can help them manage difficult feelings and calm down.[19] Imagine how you might feel if your partner refused to look at you when you felt distressed. Contrast this with how you would feel if your partner looked into your eyes with compassion and concern. Babies draw the same comfort and connection from loving eye contact. (Of course, if you're anxious or angry when trying to put your baby to sleep, you may want to avoid eye contact until you settle down; otherwise he or she will pick up on these feelings when looking into your eyes.)

Parents who follow the advice to avoid eye contact at sleep time—no matter how upset their babies become—are occasionally distraught to find that their children begin to refuse to make eye contact with them at any time. For parents, this is hugely upsetting—and in this situation they need to sensitively and persistently attempt to re-engage their babies and help them feel secure.

All about Naps

Parents often encounter difficulties at nap time; their babies may take a long time to fall asleep, wake up grumpy, or not nap at all. Also, like nighttime sleep, parents receive all sorts of nonfactual information about what babies need; for instance, that they should be awake for two hours and then asleep for two hours ("two hours up, two hours down"). Babies tend to develop patterns of naps for a while (for example, a baby might take two longer naps and one shorter one each day), but these patterns change over time and vary from child to child. Figuring out what babies need for naps is a matter of reading them well. The key is to wait for their tired signs before settling them down for sleep. Babies who wake up happy and ready to go have had enough sleep (even if it was just a thirty-minute nap); babies who are fussy are giving you a cue to settle them back to sleep. If you know they will wake up grumpy, feeding or patting them just before they normally wake can help them sleep longer.

It's also necessary to be sensitive to your baby's personality. Anni's son Zac would sleep anywhere if he was tired—at lectures, cafés, or friends' houses—so she didn't worry at all about his nap routine. Her other boys, however, napped better at home, so it didn't work for Anni to go out just before they needed a nap.

Finally, there's the tricky question of whether or not to cancel the late nap. As babies get older, their last nap of the day can start to interfere with bedtime—in other words, if they take a nap at four in the afternoon, they won't be ready to go to bed again until much later that night. However, if they don't take an afternoon nap, they can become whiny and grumpy in the early evening. This transition period is common: The best way to get through it is to make an easy, quick dinner and schedule bedtime (and the bedtime routine) earlier. After a month or so, babies adjust to these changes.

Gentle Techniques for Specific Age Groups

Getting babies to sleep may involve gentle patting, rubbing, singing, rocking, storytelling, or lying quietly next to them. Some parents enjoy helping their children go to sleep, and others prefer a less hands-on method (for example, Anni's oldest son Zac used to fall asleep listening to story tapes). The following are some settling ideas from other parents:

> I've fed [my babies] to sleep when it worked, which was about 99 percent of the time, until they were about two. When it didn't work, I'd either jog around with the baby in my arms or pat her bottom and sing to her. I liked this one, because my singing was a cue to her to stop the grizzle [fussing] and sleep.

> Giving babies lots of loving touch or a massage can help them feel safe, secure, and sleepy. Massage them a couple of times a week or just before bed as part of the bedtime routine.

> We hugged them and told them what we were going to do [while they slept]; for example, "It's time for a rest, and when you wake up, we will come and get you straightaway; we are only folding washing [laundry] or vacuuming" (mentioning something unexciting usually works). Sometimes we had to sit in the room for a minute until they settled down.

> Rocking and singing worked for the first ten to twelve months, and then I would lie down with her and rock or pat her. She sometimes fell asleep in the pram [stroller]. Nothing else worked because she had reflux and needed to sleep upright. Now I lie down with her and pretend to sleep.

In this next section, we give some suggestions of how to settle babies at different ages. The key is to do what works for you and your little one. Most of these methods work for some babies some of the time! If you want to modify your routine, see later in this chapter for ways to gently change sleep techniques.

Birth to Eight Weeks

Try to learn your babies' tired signs and help them go to sleep as soon as you notice, before they become too upset. If you delay putting them to bed, they can become overtired and find it more difficult to fall asleep (which can be very frustrating for you both!).

Getting newborns to sleep usually involves holding and rocking (for example, in a baby sling or a rocking chair), which helps comfort them as they slowly adjust to being in the world. It is also completely natural for babies to fall asleep feeding (have you ever watched other baby mammals?). If you're breast-feeding and thinking about using a pacifier, it's best to wait until after breast-feeding is well established— usually about six to eight weeks.

Some babies are happy to drift off to sleep in their cribs if you put them to bed awake sometimes—or even all of the time—but others need more movement and assistance. Swaddling infants before sleep helps them feel secure (and stops them from waking themselves up with jerky arm movements). Firmly wrap a large piece of light-weight cloth or soft blanket around your baby, but remember not to wrap him too tightly or in too many layers because overheating has been linked with SIDS.

Help babies gradually sleep longer at night by supporting the development of their "day/night" circadian rhythm: clearly distinguish day from night by allowing them to sleep in their bedrooms in normal light during the day and by dimming the lights and reducing noise and activity levels at night.

Two to Five Months

Continue to look for your babies' tired signs, and put them to bed as soon as possible. Many infants in this age group still like to be rocked to sleep, while others prefer being rocked for a while and then being placed in their cribs and cuddled or patted to sleep. Some babies no longer need rocking and can go to sleep by themselves when you place them in their cribs and give them a little pat.

Breast-feeding babies to sleep is still fine, if you are comfortable with it. Some mothers happily breast-feed their babies to sleep until they are weaned; however, some babies who are used to this bedtime routine will refuse to go to sleep with anyone except Mom! So you might want to give them opportunities to fall asleep in different ways so other people can settle them down too.

This is a great age to start setting up simple sleep cues, as we discussed earlier: swaddling, listening to a CD or singing a lullaby, or sitting in a rocking chair. At night, sleep cues might also include a relaxing bath and massage or books.

Five to Twelve Months

Everything mentioned for younger babies also applies to babies in this age group. Consider gently changing any sleep techniques that aren't working now that your child is older and more mature. Many babies are happy to be patted to sleep, which is helpful as they get heavier. Although many parents enjoy cuddling their babies to sleep, you might want to set up some sleep cues to help them go to sleep without you when you're ready for that step.

Twelve to Eighteen Months

Continue with your day and night bedtime routines. At this age, children often like to cuddle or lie near you as they fall asleep. Keep this up as long as you are happy to do so. If you start to resent it, though, then it's time to ease yourself out of the picture. One technique is to sit in a chair and read a book while your baby falls asleep (a book light can help you read in a dark room). Gradually begin to slip out of the room now and then, saying, "I'll be back in a minute, honey"—but make sure you do come back! Eventually you will be able to reassure them from the next room. Remember to be flexible, though. It's not uncommon for children to again need a parent after they have been putting themselves to sleep for a while, especially if they have difficult days or need extra comfort and reassurance for another reason.

Eighteen Months and Older

At this age, some children enjoy listening to a story as a nighttime routine, and many still like Mom or Dad to sit or lie down with them. These bedtime cuddles can be particularly delicious, but if you're ready to change the routine, most children will cope if the transition happens gradually and if you are sensitive to their need for extra cuddles or time. Story or music CDs and a night-light can help children at this age go to sleep without you.

Revisit and Adapt Your Sleep Techniques

At some point, you will probably want to change your sleep techniques, perhaps because someone else will be caring for your child (and that person can't feed or rock a baby, for instance). Sleep techniques also become less effective over time or because you are tired of the routine (for example, if you no longer want to feed your baby or he becomes too heavy to rock). Anne Kohn explains the following to parents:

> You can't treat a newborn in the way you treat a one-year-old, so you need to change what you do at each age and stage of development. If parents are tired of rocking their seven-month-old baby to sleep, for example, they may say to me, "I've done the wrong thing." I say, "You haven't done the wrong thing, it's just a matter of going down a different path now."

This mother of four puts it another way:

> You won't "spoil" your baby by practicing a certain sleep technique. Just because you let your baby share your bed for the first few months doesn't mean that [he or she] will be sleeping

there for the next twenty years! Whenever you decide [your sleep technique] needs to change, you can work toward changing it.

Whether you want to change babies' sleep associations, move them into their own cribs or beds, help them put themselves to sleep, or help them sleep for longer periods, you need to see things from your baby's perspective for a gentle transition. When thinking about making changes, keep these guiding principles in mind:

- Children should always fall asleep feeling that all is well with the world;[20] they should know that someone who loves them will be there if needed.[21]

- Try to get some sleep yourself—it will be easier to implement changes if you feel relaxed and well rested.

- Change takes time; you need to proceed at your baby's pace.

- Look to your baby for feedback—can she manage the changes?

These principles are well illustrated in the following advice from parenting writers Martha and William Pieper:

> If you offer your baby relationship pleasure rather than relationship deprivation, you will help him go to sleep secure in the conviction that you love him and want him to be happy.
>
> Although in the first year you may have to return many times to your baby's crib to rock him, give him the breast or bottle, or stroke him, your baby will learn both that you can be relied on to respond to his needs and also that he can put himself to sleep in a contented manner (and not out of despair). Over time, as your baby learns that his cries will be responded to, he will need less input from you to feel comforted and sleep.[22]

Marianne Nicholson adds this word of advice:

> It's so important for parents to understand that change is something that is negotiated in the relationship with their baby. It's important to talk to the baby if you're trying to implement

some change. The baby won't understand what's being said, but will pick up on the tone.

Change Your Baby's Sleep Associations

Change needs to be gradual and gentle; abrupt shifts in babies' sleep associations will likely cause upset. For example, if you would like your older baby to start falling asleep without the breast, you could feed her and then gently take her off the breast awake, rocking her in your arms or patting her in the crib. If she protests, begin breast-feeding again, then take her off and try again. She may end up falling asleep on the breast the first few times, but persistence over days or weeks will eventually result in a new sleep technique.

Rocking is one technique that works well for little babies but can become tiresome as they get heavier. Anne Kohn has the following suggestion for parents in this situation:

> Babies' sleep cycles are usually more established by the time they are around four months old. So if parents want to begin weaning them off rocking, they can tire them out during play-time by amping up the physical activity (which they're usually ready for at that stage). For example, they can give baby tummy time (although not all babies like this), rolling games, and so on. It can be a really fun and interactive time.
>
> Babies may still need to be rocked, but it takes less time because they're ready for sleep. Gradually wean them from being rocked by rocking for five minutes to slow them down and then putting them in their cots [cribs] when they're drowsy. Depending on temperament, some babies may still need to be asleep, while you can put other babies to bed drowsy and pat them.

This mother explains how she gently changed her baby's sleep association:

> Initially Ella would only go to sleep while I was holding and walking her. [When she was older,] I would put her into the

nest [baby sleep hammock] awake and cradle her with my body and rock her. I gradually moved my body farther away until I had my hand on her. Then I would put her in and rock the nest from the outside [without touching her], and eventually I would put her in and she would go to sleep herself. This took weeks though, and I would only try a new variation on the first sleep of the day, reverting back to the original methods as the day progressed. She could put herself to sleep at four months.

Similarly, this mother was able to help her baby learn to sleep more independently by gradual transition:

I waited until my daughter was about four months old; she was always fed or rocked to sleep, then I started putting her down when drowsy and staying with her while patting, singing, and stroking her head until she went to sleep. Sometimes I had to pick her up if she was grizzling [fussing] a bit, but when she stopped, I put her back down again. After about four days, I could pop her into bed and leave the room, [and] she drifted off to sleep all by herself. Sometimes I needed to go in and tell her "Ssshhhh, Mommy's here," and she would nod off with just a bit of reassurance.

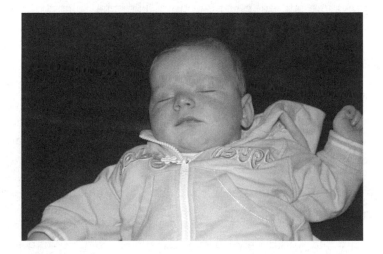

Are There Good and Bad Sleep Associations?

In the world of baby sleep advice, some sleep associations are considered to be bad (for example, a mother's breast, sucking on a pacifier, or being rocked or comforted to sleep), while others are said to be good (such as a cuddly toy, swaddling, or using a crib).

The essential difference between good and bad sleep associations is that those considered *good* do not involve a parent. It is thought that when babies get used to these associations, they will no longer call out for their parents when they wake at night. There is nothing wrong with this theory, and there is nothing wrong with gently working toward helping your baby develop sleep associations that don't involve you—if you want to and if your child shows signs that he or she is ready. There is also nothing wrong with any of the so-called *bad* sleep associations if you and your baby are happy. These associations are often discouraged because of the mistaken belief that once you help children go to sleep, they will always need your help to do so. You can relax—there is no urgent need for them to learn to sleep without you! Babies often grow out of sleep associations, and if they don't, some persistent parental assistance can help them on their way, as the following story about Noah illustrates:

> **Birth to three months:** We rocked Noah to sleep in our arms until he was approximately three months old.
>
> **Three to twelve months:** From three months on, we put him in his cot [crib], which was next to our bed, and held his hand until he slept. We gradually shortened the time we held his hand and started leaving the room when he wasn't quite asleep; eventually we could leave him wide awake but very happy to doze off by himself.
>
> When Noah started rolling over in bed at eight months, we let him roll around for five to ten minutes to wind down, then rubbed his back until he slept. It took a month or so of this until he learned how to sleep on his own again.

Twelve to eighteen months: When he was twelve months old and learning how to stand up in bed, it coincided with him dropping from two sleeps [naps] to one. Since his middle-of-the-day breast-feed coincided with his sleep time, I fed him to sleep. He also moved in to his own room at this age, which he loved from day one.

At fifteen months, I dropped the midday feed. I did the bedtime routine (diaper change, read two books, then lie down next to him on our bed) and transferred him to his cot after he fell asleep.

Eighteen months and up: At eighteen months, I started putting him in his cot with his favorite soft toy. [His father or I] then lay down on the floor next to the cot and held his hand until he fell asleep. After a month or so of this, I could put him in bed and leave the room. He would then go to sleep by himself.

The settling needs of most babies are dynamic—what works one month may not work the next. Parents can also get tired of particular routines and seek to modify what they do at bedtime or nap time. Fortunately, babies are amenable to change that is slow and respectful. Of course, settling is only part of the picture—there is also staying asleep. In the next chapter, we look at addressing some common sleep problems that keep babies and their parents awake.

Key Points

- Babies usually need their parents' assistance to settle down for sleep; recognizing their tired signs and developing a baby-friendly sleep routine will help both babies and parents.

- Stay as calm as possible at sleep time—this will increase your chances of helping your baby settle.

- Different settling techniques work for different babies.

- Wherever your baby sleeps, make sure he or she sleeps safely.

- Parents can expect to use a variety of settling techniques as their babies get older.

- Over time, most parents want to change the way they help their babies sleep, and there are gentle techniques to do so.

NOTES

1. Stanley Greenspan, with Nancy Breslau Lewis, *Building Healthy Minds: The Six Experiences that Create Intelligence and Emotional Growth in Babies and Young Children* (New York: Perseus, 1999), 368.

2. Harriet Hiscock and Melissa Wake, "Randomised Controlled Trial of Behavioural Infant Sleep Intervention to Improve Infant Sleep and Maternal Mood," *British Medical Journal* 324 (May 2002): 1062.

3. All Nicholson and Kohn quotes: Marianne Nicholson, interview, February 9, 2006; and Anne Kohn, interview, March 20, 2006.

4. For example, Gina Ford, *The New Contented Little Baby Book: The Secret to Calm and Confident Parenting from One of the World's Top Maternity Nurses* (London: Vermilion, 2002); and Tizzie Hall, *Save Our Sleep: A Parents' Guide toward Happy, Sleeping Babies* (Melbourne, Australia: Pan Macmillan, 2006).

5. Many books that advocate rigid breast-feeding schedules can set up mothers for frustration and failure; this advice is unfair to both mothers and babies. Introducing formula early, feeding young infants from bottles, and breast-feeding according to the clock—rather than a baby's needs—can all detrimentally affect a mother's ability to produce enough milk and a baby's ability to firmly attach to the nipple. Specialist breast-feeding books, such as *Breastfeeding with Confidence: A Do-It-Yourself Guide* by Sue Cox (Sydney: Finch, 2004), and specialist breast-feeding organizations, such as La Leche League, provide accurate information and support. Visit www.lllusa.org to find out more.

6. American Academy of Pediatrics, policy statement, "Breastfeeding and the Use of Human Milk," http://aappolicy.aappublications.org/cgi/content/full/pediatrics;115/2/496 (accessed July 2006); Pat Thomas, "Suck on This," *The Ecologist* (April 2006): 22–33; and Australian National Health and Medical

Research Council, "Dietary Guidelines for Children and Adolescents in Australia, Incorporating the Infant Feeding Guidelines for Health Workers Endorsed 10 April 2003" (July 2, 2003), www.nhmrc.gov.au/publications/synopses/_files/n34.pdf (accessed October 2006). For further reading, refer to "101 Reasons to Breastfeed Your Child," www.breastfeed.com/resources/articles/101reasonsp1.htm.

7. Jon Weimer, *The Economic Benefits of Breast Feeding: A Review and Analysis*, Food Assistance and Nutrition Research Report No. 13, Food and Rural Economics Division, Economic Research Service, U.S. Department of Agriculture, Washington, D.C., 2001; and Thomas M. Ball and Anne L. Wright, "Health Care Costs of Formula-Feeding in the First Year of Life," *Pediatrics* 103, no. 4 (1999): 870–876, as cited in the American Academy of Pediatrics, policy statement, "Breastfeeding and the Use of Human Milk" (accessed July 2006).

8. Jeanne Raisler, Cheryl Alexander, and Patricia O'Campo, "Breast-feeding and Infant Illness: A Dose-Response Relationship?" *American Journal of Public Health* 89, no. 1 (January 1999): 25–30.

9. Australian National Health and Medical Research Council, "Dietary Guidelines for Children and Adolescents" (July 2, 2003) (accessed October 2006).

10. Yvette O'Dowd, "Just Breastmilk, Thanks!" Australian Breastfeeding Association, www.breastfeeding.asn.au/bfinfo/justbm.html (accessed October 2006). For good guidelines on when to introduce solid foods, see "Feeding Infants and Toddlers: Starting Solid Foods," www.askdrsears.com/html/3/T032000.asp.

11. See note 9 above.

12. San Diego County Breastfeeding Coalition, "Breastfeeding Facts," www.breastfeeding.org/bfacts/bottle.html (accessed July 2006).

13. Margot Sunderland, *The Science of Parenting: Practical Guidance on Sleep, Crying, Play and Building Emotional Wellbeing for Life* (London: Dorling Kindersley, 2006), 67.

14. More benefits of co-sleeping are detailed in Pinky McKay, *Sleeping Like a Baby: Simple Sleep Solutions for Infants and Toddlers* (Melbourne, Australia: Penguin, 2006); and Sunderland, *The Science of Parenting*.

15. These guidelines have been adapted from the following sources: Howard Chilton, *Baby on Board: Understanding What Your Baby Needs* (Sydney: Finch, 2003), 108–111; "Is Your Baby Sleeping Safely?" pamphlet produced by Australian Breastfeeding Association, Baby Friendly Hospital Initiative Australia, Maternity Coalition, Midwives in Independent Practice, and Australian Lactation Consultants' Association (2004); Central Sydney Area Health Service, "Early Childhood Health Service Guidelines on Settling for Health Professionals," *Australian Association for Infant Mental Health Newsletter* 15, no. 1 (March 2003): 10–11; and McKay, *Sleeping Like a Baby*, 72.

16. National SIDS Council of Australia, "SIDS & Kids: Safe Sleeping," www.sidsandkids.org/documents/safesleepbro_000.pdf; and McKay, *Sleeping Like a Baby*.

17. Peter J. Fleming, Peter S. Blair, Christopher Bacon, and Peter J. Berry, eds., *Sudden Unexpected Death in Infancy: The CESDI SUDI Studies 1993–1996* (London: The Stationery Office, 2000).

18. Li I. Zhang, Shaowen Bao, and Michael M. Merzenich, "Disruption of Primary Auditory Cortex by Synchronous Auditory Inputs during a Critical Period," *Proceedings of the National Academy of Sciences of the United States of America* 99, no. 4 (February 2002): 2309–2314.

19. Sue Gerhardt, *Why Love Matters: How Affection Shapes a Baby's Brain* (New York: Brunner-Routledge, 2004).

20. Sunderland, *The Science of Parenting*.

21. Central Sydney Area Health Service, "Early Childhood Health Service Guidelines," 10.

22. Martha and William Pieper, www.babycenter.com (accessed October 2006).

CHAPTER 6

Common Sleep Problems—and How to Cope with Them

*As you make any changes, it is wise to remember the mantra
"gradually with love" and make each change in baby steps.[1]*
PINKY MCKAY

In the previous chapter we detailed gentle approaches to help your baby settle down and sleep. But some infants can be extremely hard to settle and others wake up a lot. For example, Anni's baby Ben sometimes woke up eight times a night and could take an hour to settle back to sleep. Other babies have different sleep issues: Maybe your child takes forever to go to sleep, wakes up every hour to feed, or wakes up at 2 A.M. and won't go back to sleep. This chapter provides advice on common sleep problems that babies (and therefore their parents!) experience—whether the reason is physical, emotional, behavioral, or all three.

When it comes to dealing with sleep problems, whatever the cause, the major difficulty is that babies who wake up a lot have *very* tired parents. Being exhausted makes it hard to remember what day it is, let alone develop a methodical plan to figure out what is troubling your baby and how to resolve it. If this sounds like you, this chapter gives you some possibilities to consider—both for infants and toddlers who have started waking recently and those who have longer-term waking issues. Anni wishes that someone had given her this kind of advice when she was trying to determine what was wrong with Ben. It took years of resolute effort to discover that Ben reacted to chemicals in food and that even healthy foods such as watermelon or tuna could dramatically affect his sleep.

Do We Really Have a Sleep Problem?

Before embarking on this problem-solving venture, we recommend that you ask yourself the question we raised in chapter 1: Is the night waking normal? Wanting to be close to parents at night is just normal infant behavior—fixing this "sleep problem" could be as easy as having your baby sleep on a mattress next to yours or in your bed, if that works for you (see pages 114 to 116 for safe sleeping and bed-sharing instructions). Also, as we've shown in other chapters, many guidelines as to how babies "should" sleep are fabricated by the authors—they are neither based on credible evidence nor on the needs of your individual baby. Furthermore, strictly following these guidelines can actually cause sleep problems, as researchers in a Swiss sleep study involving 493 children found: "Unrealistic or rigid parental expectations of sleep need without taking the child's age into account have been shown to be a significant cause for bedtime difficulties and for frequent night and/or early morning wakings."[2] Remember, too, that in many cultures no one puts the baby to bed—babies fall asleep with the family in the midst of different activities. These children are not considered to have a "sleep problem" and still learn to put themselves to sleep just fine.

Another false "sleep problem" could be one that *you* cause! Sometimes highly responsive parents can inadvertently create environments that lead to frequent or unnecessary waking. While we encourage all parents to respond to their babies' needs, some parents tend to their babies more than necessary. For example, they rush to check on or feed their babies with every little fuss they make during sleep time. But, according to Marianne Nicholson, former child and family nurse practitioner, "If baby is waking up, sometimes he'll need you to help go back to sleep and sometimes he won't. Wait until baby calls you and says, 'I'm not managing this, I need some help.' That doesn't mean he's going to cry loudly, but don't rush anxiously to your baby unless he needs you." Parenting educator and writer Elizabeth Pantley shares similar advice, suggesting that parents learn "the difference between sleeping noises and awake noises": "When Baby makes a noise, stop. Listen. Wait. Peek. As you listen attentively to her noises and watch her, you will learn the difference between sleeping snorts and 'I'm waking up and I need you now' noises."[3]

Physical and Emotional Problems That Cause Wakefulness

A wide range of problems can cause babies pain or irritation or make them more sensitive and wakeful. In this section, we discuss the most common physical and emotional reasons for wakefulness. If your baby does have sleep problems, we recommend first considering the following issues—and either rule them out or take steps to help your baby feel better.

Difficult Birth

Prolonged or difficult births can cause infants to be unsettled; those who were born in an abnormal position (for example, posterior, breech, shoulder, or face presentation), with the help of forceps or suction, or by cesarean section are more susceptible to sleep problems than those born without complications. This is because a physically traumatic birth can cause a misalignment of the baby's skeletal framework, leading to possible muscular spasms, pain, and discomfort. A cranial osteopath, pediatric osteopath, or chiropractor who has experience working with babies is always worth seeing in these cases—and they can sometimes perform miracles.

Exposure to Harmful Substances In Utero

Babies who have been exposed regularly to nicotine, alcohol, or other harmful drugs in utero can be more irritable and reactive to stress (they also experience a wide range of other health problems). They may have become addicted to the substance and undergo the effects of withdrawal. Harmful drugs can easily disrupt babies' immature brain chemistry and bodily rhythms (such as heart rate), making them more difficult to settle. If you think this could be an issue, look for a nonjudgmental health professional to give you advice.

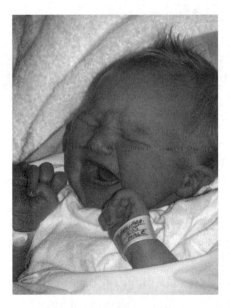

Colic

This is a condition in which otherwise healthy babies scream inconsolably for long periods of time for no identifiable reason. Feeding, rocking, and other soothing methods can have little or no impact. Colic can last for a few weeks, and it usually clears up by twelve weeks. It is just awful for parents and babies—see the following two pages for tips on dealing with this distressing problem.

Dealing with Colic

Colicky babies are very hard to care for, and their inconsolable crying can drive parents to despair. First we recommend that you systematically seek professional help to determine the cause of the problem and how you can best cope with it. While you are figuring it out, you especially need to have a good support plan in place for yourself (see chapter 8). Ideally this will involve you and your partner supporting each other and your baby rather than resorting to blame or avoidance.

Mothers and fathers of colicky infants frequently have high stress levels—no matter what they try, they cannot help their babies calm down. Because these babies are very sensitive, they can hear tension in their parents' voices and see it in their faces, and this can make them more upset, thereby perpetuating a negative cycle of stress. When dealing with your colicky baby while he's upset (no matter how tense you may feel on the inside), do your best to maintain a calm, soothing voice and facial expression around him (see chapter 5 for some tips to settle down yourself).

During the periods between crying (as short as they may be) you can often do fruitful work to help colicky babies develop a stronger connection with you and feel more secure in their environment. When you initiate interactions—for example, smile at or talk to your baby—consciously take time to wait for her reaction. This lets you practice slowing down and tuning in to your baby, and gives you both a chance to enjoy each other. When your baby smiles or makes a happy sound, immediately reinforce this behavior by imitating it, then wait again and allow her to respond. Mirroring babies' faces and sounds helps them become aware of their happy feelings.

In your day-to-day activities, practice using a warm and confident tone of voice to describe what is happening for her.[4] For example, "We're going to change your diaper now, Catherine. I'm laying you on your changing table, and see—here's your diaper, and I'm undoing the buttons on your pants." Talking to babies this way encourages them to feel connected to you and to what is happening, and seeing your loving face and hearing your confident tone can reassure them that all is right with the world.

Working with babies in this way when they are not crying is unlikely to change matters immediately. But if you incorporate these practices into your daily interactions with your children, you can help them begin to feel that life has predictable patterns and that they are in a loving, calm environment.

Many parents of colicky babies understandably lose confidence in their settling techniques and often quickly move from one method to another in desperate attempts to settle them. Establishing a sleep routine for a frantically screaming infant can seem impossible; however, not having a set routine can sometimes make babies unsure of what to expect next, making them even more difficult to settle down. So do your best to calmly continue with your settling technique at bedtime or nap time. For example, if you use Harvey Karp's techniques (see page 199 for details), try them for at least a couple of weeks.

Teething

The arrival of teeth is a major reason for wakefulness—and can go on for months and months for some infants. Many babies begin teething at around four or five months of age, but (as with all aspects of development) some begin earlier and some later. The signs of teething are usually dribbling, red cheeks, chewing, cheek rubbing, irritability, and oral pain. At night, the main relief you can provide is teething gel or infant pain relievers (follow the guidelines carefully) and extra cuddles.

Sick or Recently Immunized

Illness and immunization can cause babies to become temporarily more wakeful. If you think your child might be sick and you're not sure with what, schedule a checkup with your pediatrician. Ear infections in particular can make babies wake up screaming—but can be hard for parents to identify.

Environmental Irritants or Discomfort

Modern homes can contain lots of potential irritants. Make sure that the place in which your baby sleeps is free from dust, mold, and cigarette smoke: Some babies are very sensitive to small dust particles or mold spores. Also check for annoying visitors such as mosquitoes, fleas, mites, and pinworms. Make sure babies aren't too cold or hot at night (baby sleeping bags can help keep them warm and a fan can help keep the room cool). Also ensure that clothes or bedding are not irritating.

Hidden Physical Problems

If none of the above issues explain your baby's wakefulness, it is worth checking for hidden physical problems. Ask your pediatrician to thoroughly examine your baby, looking for signs of reflux, ear infection, food or environmental allergies, sleep apnea, and other illnesses or irritations. Follow his or her advice about how best to address these problems—it may involve medication or a formula change (if you are not breast-feeding). In rare instances, breast milk itself may be the cause of your baby's health condition, yet in this case changing your diet to address food intolerances often helps (see next page). If your pediatrician or other health professional advises you to stop breast-feeding, we recommend that you consult a qualified lactation specialist for a second opinion.

Food Intolerances

Finally, after your baby is medically checked over, you should consider the possibility that he or she might have food intolerances. Reactions to food, formula, or food consumed by a breast-feeding mother can seriously disrupt babies' sleep and make them generally colicky, cranky, and unsettled. A website dedicated to helping parents with this topic is www.fedupwithfoodadditives.info. You may want to try the suggested elimination diet if you are breast-feeding or a change of formula if applicable (under medical guidance). Addressing food intolerances can be enormously beneficial for some babies.

Emotional Upsets

Babies are very sensitive to changes in their emotional environments, particularly in their parents' emotional states. Stressful events such as parents separating, parents arguing or dealing with emotional shocks, the arrival of new siblings, starting day care, or moving can all affect how babies feel. Also be mindful of separation anxiety. When change occurs, such as Mom going back to work, babies can wake up more often looking for reassurance that their mothers are still there. Even positive changes, such as taking a vacation, can often make them wake more than usual. Generally babies need comfort, sensitivity, and extra cuddles until the stressful situation passes. If the wakefulness persists longer than a month, try some of the suggestions in the "Techniques for Addressing the Most Sleep Common Problems" section (pages 142–150).

Trauma

Babies and young children who have been traumatized can find it very difficult to go to sleep and may wake repeatedly at night. This trauma may arise from a single event, a series of connected events, or chronic, enduring stress.[5] Triggers for trauma can include abuse or neglect, witnessing or being the victim of violence, extended separations from a primary caregiver, or invasive and painful medical procedures. Children can recover from trauma with the help of a warm and responsive caregiver who makes them feel safe and secure. However, if you feel your child's sleep problems may be the result of unresolved trauma, seek the assistance of a skilled child mental health specialist.

Seeking Further Assistance

When it comes to wakefulness with physical or emotional causes, you can address many problems quite easily—and some clear thinking about new ways of doing things can help your baby sleep better. Parents are most likely to find the longer-term issues, hidden physical conditions, or sensitivities the most difficult to resolve. If you and your doctor, pediatrician, or nurse practitioner can figure out the nature of the problem, that is a good start. You can begin investigating ways to help your baby as well as gain some idea of how long it is likely to last.

Doctors occasionally tell parents, "Your baby is healthy—there is nothing wrong with him." Often the "healthy baby" diagnosis means that the doctor doesn't know why your baby is waking up so much. In this case, we recommend that you get a second, third, or fourth opinion. Also, if the problem is one in which the doctor has no expertise, such as food sensitivities or silent reflux, you may need to see a different type of health professional or a specialist—such as a dietician or food allergy specialist. Some parents also find that alternative health practitioners such as osteopaths, chiropractors, naturopaths, or homeopaths can be very helpful. The key with these professionals is to ensure that they have experience dealing with babies and also with your baby's specific problem.

Techniques for Addressing the Most Common Sleep Problems

Addressing sleep difficulties starts with looking at physical and emotional disturbances and either resolving them or ruling them out as the underlying cause. It also involves setting up certain preconditions for sleep such as a sleep-time routine, sufficient physical activity and naps, and ensuring your baby has enough to eat. If you've done all this and your baby is still having trouble sleeping, it's time to begin directly tackling whatever isn't working. The following section gives advice for coping with the most common sleep problems. Gently changing babies' sleep patterns and helping them overcome these issues usually takes time and patience. Once you make a plan, we recommend that you stick with it for at least a couple of weeks to give it time to work (unless your baby gives you clear signals that he really doesn't like it).

Baby Takes a Long Time to Fall Asleep

If babies take a long time to fall asleep, first ask yourself whether they are really tired; you may be putting them to bed too early. If you think this might be the case, watch for tired signs and try a later bedtime. For older babies, you can also try giving them lots of activity every

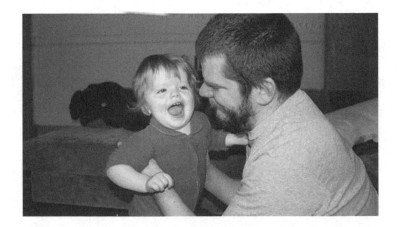

afternoon—rolling, climbing, throwing, and running—so they are physically worn out at the end of the day.

If they still take a long time to fall asleep but you're sure they are indeed tired, they may need a longer wind-down time. Remember to make your house unexciting at bedtime—turn off the TV, dim the lights, make everything quiet—and extend the routine a little, perhaps with a few extra books, a story, a massage, or a longer bath. Remember, too, to relax yourself; babies can find it more difficult to settle if you feel stressed. You might want to unwind by taking a bath together or listening to soft music while you get your baby ready for bed. Sometimes children have trouble going to sleep if they are chemically overstimulated. Make sure that they don't drink soda or sugary drinks, and if you're breast-feeding, consider reducing your intake of caffeine and other stimulants.

For babies who attend day care, ask yourself whether you've been able to spend enough time connecting between pickup time and bedtime. If not, think of ways to do this, such as playing on the floor for a half hour after dinner and before you start your nighttime routine. They likely missed you during the day, and they need to feel close to you. Taking a while to go to sleep may be their way of spending time with the people they love most in the world!

Baby Wakes Every Hour to Feed or Use a Pacifier (More than Four to Six Months Old)

Babies who frequently wake at night to feed or suck on a pacifier are really hard work. Parents can usually cope with a few days or so of continual waking, but after a while, it leaves them exhausted and frustrated. Fortunately, you can avoid this problem or reduce night waking in a number of ways.

First, you need to eliminate physical or emotional upsets that could cause this behavior. Read through the issues discussed earlier in this chapter, and see if addressing any of them helps. At the same time, work on sleep preparation—use a gentle bedtime routine (see chapter 5) and make sure your baby goes to bed tired. If you are co-sleeping, try moving your baby a little farther away from you; for example, in a crib a few feet from your bed or in a sidecar arrangement. This way babies are less likely to smell you when they rouse from a deep sleep and may wake up less frequently.

Changing the sleep/wake patterns of your baby can also help. This method is called "scheduled awakenings." It is as clinically effective as "sleep training," but a far gentler way of reducing night waking.[6] Record the times your baby usually wakes, and then over the following nights, wake her up 15 to 30 minutes before she would normally wake to feed or call for you. Resettle her without feeding (if you can) or feed her if she is hungry or won't settle. For the first few nights to a week, your baby will most likely wake up as usual, but (if the technique is working) will eventually sleep through the time she would normally wake. Once she starts to do so, you can stop the scheduled awakening.

You can also try modifying your baby's suck/sleep association. Elizabeth Pantley has a lot of good information on this method; in essence, her advice is to gently change the association between sucking on the breast and sleep. Bit by bit, you can help your baby become used to falling asleep without sucking: when breast-feeding before or during sleep time, remove the nipple, wait, reinsert, and remove again. If this is an issue for you, we recommend Elizabeth Pantley's book The No-Cry Sleep Solution and website (see page 199 for details).

Breast-feeding to sleep is one of nature's gifts, and babies will naturally fall asleep on the breast (or bottle) when they are very little. But to avoid complete reliance on this technique (or sucking on a pacifier), when your baby is tired and full of milk, consistently try other ways of getting him to sleep, such as rocking or patting or taking him for a long walk in the baby sling or stroller. Also, from early on, regularly hand him over to your partner to keep his or her settling skills up to date!

Some parents find that babies sleep longer if they have an additional late feed. As you go to bed yourself, give your baby a "roll over" feed if possible—tanking up at night can keep some infants asleep longer.

Baby Wakes Frequently for Comfort (More than Six Months Old)

If your baby wakes up frequently and doesn't want to feed but needs a lot of comforting to go back to sleep, first look through the possible physical and emotional difficulties discussed earlier in this chapter. Frequent waking is often caused by some disturbance in your baby's life, so be sure to rule out all potential problems. If you have eliminated these causes, one option is to live with it for another week or two. Some issues will resolve themselves over time.

Another way of managing this situation is to keep things dark, boring, and simple when babies wake at night. Don't hype them up or play with them; just gently try to resettle them. You could also include music as a sleep cue: if you haven't already, make music part of your sleep routine, and then leave it on all night or play it when babies wake up, which may help them resettle easily. The "scheduled awakenings" method can also help to change sleep associations (see opposite page).

Many parents also find that babies wake frequently because they miss them at night—some infants simply sleep better near Mom and Dad. If you think this might be the case, try bringing your baby into your room or into bed with you (see pages 115 to 116 for safe bed-sharing guidelines). Alternatively, you can set up a cot or mattress in your baby's room, and with your partner, take turns sleeping on it. This allows babies to have the company they desire, and one parent gets a relatively undisturbed night's sleep. These options really work for some families because babies have been waking up simply because they want to be close to their parents.

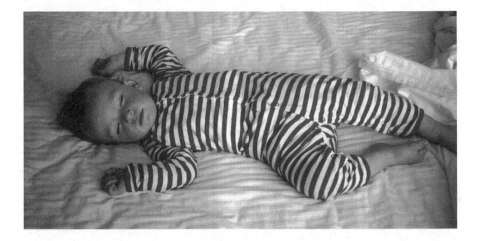

Baby Only Lets One Parent Put Him or Her to Sleep

While some babies will happily let anyone put them to bed, others are very attached to being put to sleep by only Mom or only Dad. Avoid this problem from early on by making sure your partner or another caregiver (if appropriate) takes turns putting your baby to sleep. Let them develop their own settling methods; it probably took you a while to figure out how best to settle your child, so give them a chance before imposing your routine. Their settling technique might be completely different from what you do; for example, going for a walk in the sling, rocking in the rocking chair, or cuddling in bed (and the more successful settling methods you have, the better!).

If someone new will be settling your baby, say Dad or a relative who is going to take over a couple of nights a week, have this person spend lots of quality time with your child before attempting to settle him or her to sleep. Give babies lots of positive encouragement to help them feel safe and secure with this person. You may want to then have the caregiver gradually become part of the pre-bed routine, before eventually taking over from you. When making this transition, make sure your baby isn't overly tired or hungry. It may also be helpful to leave the house when the new caregiver is settling your baby, if your little one is likely to notice you are around or if you are tempted to interfere.

Baby Only Stays Asleep in My Arms or Lying Down Together

Many newborns (up to about three months of age) sleep best when someone holds them, and this makes sense as they are making their transition into the world. Most will start to sleep for longer periods in their cribs soon enough without too much fuss. Some older babies and toddlers, however, will suddenly begin to sleep only while being held or lying next to a parent, and wake up if Mom or Dad dares to move! Some parents don't mind this and are happy to rest or take a nap with their babies (see pages 115 to 116 for safe bed-sharing guidelines). Other parents can find this very frustrating.

If this is a problem for you, think about whether anything happened recently for your baby to need extra comfort and reassurance. Have there been a lot of changes, such as moving, parents separating, or starting day care? If you think there have, do whatever you can during awake times to help your child feel extra secure: lots of touching and holding, following a predictable rhythm, and reducing your own stress level may reassure your baby that it's okay to let you go at sleep time.

During awake times, you can also give babies lots of cues that it's safe to separate from you. Reassure them that it's all right to let you go and for them to explore, and that you will always be available to provide comfort and protection if they need it. So, if your six-month-old seems interested in a new rattle, or your fourteen-month-old wants to examine Grandma's toy box, put a positive and confident expression on your face, and say, "It's okay for you to go play with that. I'll be right here if you need me." Allow babies to play until they are ready to return to you. Then you can share in their excitement or comfort them if they become upset. If you do this repeatedly, you will give them the message that it's safe to separate from their parents, which may help them do so more easily at sleep time.

You can also try using sleep cues that don't involve you when you put your baby to bed, such as music or a teddy bear. This way, your child may not wake up when you leave because other cues are in place. Leaving your scent nearby (such as an unwashed T-shirt or nursing bra) can also help comfort babies when you are not physically present. Another idea is to make a tape of you singing nursery rhymes or softly telling a story. Get babies used to falling asleep with this tape on, and when you leave, they may not wake up because they can hear your voice.

Baby Wakes Screaming

If babies wake up screaming (rather than crying and working up to screaming), something is acutely distressing them. It is either a sudden sharp pain or a deep fear, and both require your immediate attention and reassurance. In instances where your baby is ill and you are concerned, you should seek medical advice right away. Generally, for babies who wake up screaming, it is worth scheduling a full medical checkup with your pediatrician as soon as possible, including looking for possible ear problems; this should help you ascertain whether the source is physical.

Night terrors (*pavor nocturnus*) can also cause this problem. These terrors are not nightmares but intense feelings of fear and panic. Night terrors can sometimes follow fever or periods of high stress during the day. Babies often seem to scream out in fear, but don't appear to be fully awake. Some infants can be woken to be comforted, while others will remain partially asleep and are often hard to rouse or reassure—you may need to gently restrain them to keep them from running around and harming themselves. If children have night terrors at the same time every night, wake them up fifteen minutes prior to this time and then let them drift off to sleep again. Try this method for a week to see if this helps.

Baby Wakes in the Middle of the Night, Wants to Play, and Won't Go Back to Sleep

Playful babies at night can be a nightmare! This problem can be difficult to solve, and it especially seems to be an issue for clever babies who want to keep engaging with the world (comfort yourself with this thought at 3:30 A.M.). For some infants, making things extra boring at nighttime can help. If baby is in a separate room, don't turn on any lights and don't engage with her—just try to gently settle her back to sleep. If you're sharing a room, roll over and pretend to be asleep. Other babies are just *up*—so in this case, give them some toys and books to play with in the crib or on the mattress. (If you are not planning to stay awake and observe your baby, make sure the toys are completely safe.) This can occupy some babies until they go back to sleep. Alternatively, you can go with it—some parents are night owls too, so getting up and doing something quietly until baby gets sleepy again can work.

Baby Goes to Sleep Too Late

Infants need more sleep than adults, but you may find that your baby is a night owl—you're ready for bed but your baby is still up and going. Dropping babies' late naps can help. Try keeping them awake through the last nap of the day, and see if they start getting tired earlier. You'll probably know within a week if this is effective or if the trade-off is a grumpy, overtired baby in the evening. Alternatively, you can try waking them earlier in the morning. If babies are sleeping in (say, past 7 A.M.), wake them ten minutes earlier every morning to see if this changes their sleep routine. For some parents, the best solution is to simply accept that they have a late-night baby. As long as babies get enough sleep during the day, having them stay up late can actually be fun. It can give working parents time to catch up and play with their babies, and if you have other children, it can be a nice opportunity for some one-on-one time.

Baby Wakes Too Early

Babies tend to wake up very early, so any time after 6 A.M. is definitely reasonable (you might have to start going to bed earlier!). You can also do several things to help babies get a bit more sleep in the morning. Completely darkening the room prevents early morning light from awakening them, or putting them to bed later can also be effective. To try a later bedtime, gradually move it back over a couple of weeks. Some babies, however, biologically need less sleep than others (see chapter 1). If they still wake up too early, you can leave out a stack of toys for when they wake up—some babies or toddlers will keep themselves occupied.

Baby Is Moving from the Family Bed to His or Her Own Bed

All children who start off sleeping in the family bed eventually move to their own beds or cribs—but parents can be ready for this step well before children. The key is to make the transition as gentle as possible. Placing your mattress and your baby's crib side by side often works, either in your room or baby's room.

Alternatively, some children are ready to move into their own beds or cribs—they just need the opportunity to do so. Introduce the new bed to your child and make it inviting and cozy. Have them take naps in this bed, and put them to sleep in it at bedtime. If they come into your bed at night, either leave them there (if that's okay) or return them to their bed or a mattress in your room.

Key Points

- Many difficulties can cause babies to have trouble going to sleep and to wake up more often than normal—these problems can be physical, emotional, and behavioral in nature.

- Some sleep issues are temporary, such as those caused by teething or illness, while others may require time and patience to treat, and possibly the services of a medical professional or health practitioner.

- Sleep behaviors that aren't working for parents can usually be remedied with patience and gentle changes, as long as your baby is ready. You might have to try several different approaches to find what suits you and your baby best. Keep in mind, however, that many issues will resolve themselves in time.

NOTES

1. Pinky McKay, *Sleeping Like a Baby: Simple Sleep Solutions for Infants and Toddlers* (Melbourne, Australia: Penguin, 2006), 146.

2. Ivo Iglowstein, Oskar G. Jenni, Luciano Molinari, and Remo H. Largo, "Sleep Duration from Infancy to Adolescence: Reference Values and Generational Trends," *Pediatrics* 111, no. 2 (February 2003): 302–307.

3. Elizabeth Pantley, *The No-Cry Sleep Solution: Gentle Ways to Help Your Baby Sleep Through the Night* (New York: McGraw-Hill, 2002), 133.

4. Maria Aarts, *Marte Meo: Basic Manual*, 2nd ed. (Eindhoven, Netherlands: Aarts Productions, 2008).

5. Alicia F. Lieberman and Lisa Amaya-Jackson, "Reciprocal Influences of Attachment and Trauma: Using a Dual Lens in the Assessment and Treatment of Infants, Toddlers and Preschoolers" in *Enhancing Early Attachments: Theory, Research, Intervention, and Policy*, eds. Lisa J. Berlin,

Yair Ziv, Lisa Amaya-Jackson, and Mark T. Greenberg (New York: Guilford Press, 2005), 100–124.

6. Vaughn I. Rickert and C. Merle Johnson, "Reducing Nocturnal Awakening and Crying Episodes in Infants and Young Children: A Comparison Between Scheduled Awakenings and Systematic Ignoring," *Pediatrics* 81, no. 2 (1988): 203–212.

CHAPTER 7

Responsive Parenting— Six Gifts You Can Give Your Child

Without an emotional understanding of the child, parenting skills
are of little use, and remain empty recipes that bear little
relation to the child's internal experience and needs.[1]
ARIETTA SLADE

By this point, we've explained why responsive, sensitive parenting gives children the greatest chance of growing up happy and secure. One of our many concerns with sleep training is that it requires parents to be insensitive and nonresponsive to their babies; it can numb the empathy that they have for their children's suffering. In this chapter, we explore what it means to be a responsive parent and to deal with babies' sleep needs sensitively.

Most of us know how to be an intellectual resource for our children: how to read to them, discuss issues with them, give them access to technology, and provide them with a good education. Being an emotional resource for them is more challenging and rests on six core relationship skills.[2] We like to think of the following as *gifts* you give your children through your relationship:

1. *You:* Recognize your importance to your baby.

2. *Communication:* Pay attention to what your baby is trying to tell you.

3. *Your actions:* Realize how your behavior affects your child.

4. *Empathy:* Truly understand your baby's feelings.

5. *Emotional regulation:* Manage your baby's feelings.

6. *Your feelings:* Look after your own needs.

And if babies are regularly taken care of by someone else, they need these gifts from their caregivers too!

You: Recognize Your Importance to Your Baby

Parents are the center of their baby's world: his rock, his anchor, his shining star. Babies need to know that you are there for them, attentive and attuned, especially if they are feeling powerful emotions such as fear, sadness, or anger.[3] Without your constant emotional support, they will struggle like fish out of water.

When trying to make sense of our babies' sleep-time behaviors, many parents become frustrated—and understandably so. "Why does she want me to lie down with her at bedtime? Why will my newborn only sleep for long periods in my arms? Why does she still wake at night and cry out for me?" Without comprehending how deeply babies and young children need us, this behavior can be seen as willful, naughty, or even manipulative. Yet, when we realize that babies' and children's behaviors *always* signal needs of some sort, it helps us shift our focus from the behavior to the *need* underlying the behavior.

Most parents understand that babies and young children need our guidance and support to explore their world: to find a new toy to play with when they are bored, to help them up when they fall down, and so on. When it comes to sleep, they do not stop needing us—they just need different types of help. When overwhelmed by tiredness, a baby may need comfort in the form of rocking, holding, or patting. Even if a baby or young child peacefully settles himself to sleep, he still needs his parents to stay nearby to offer reassurance and protection should the need arise. Over time, the way children need their parents at sleep time will change. For example, as newborns, Beth's boys were content to sleep in someone's arms. But just a few months later, they were happily napping alone in their bedrooms. Matthew, Beth's second baby, often settled easily in his crib when he was a few months old, but once teething began, he started needing a lot more holding and comfort. One mom found her daughter's sleep-time needs changed dramatically after her first birthday:

> Our first did not like to go to sleep alone for the entire first year of her life. However, when she was a year old, suddenly she was able to drop off by herself It was like a light switch! We didn't try any specific [new] technique, we just were doing what we'd always done: put her down awake, leave when she was calm (then go straight back in because she'd cry as soon as we left!), and creep out again once her eyes were closed.

Sensitive parenting allowed this baby to make the shift to sleeping by herself in her own time and without tears. Another mother found her son's bedtime needs changed when he started school:

> My son had been able to go to sleep by himself from about six months. When he was four, however, he began asking me to lie down with him at bedtime. This happened soon after he started school. At first I resisted, and kept insisting he go to sleep without me, but it took ages for him to settle. When I finally accepted that he just needed me at bedtime, I began to lie down with him until he went to sleep. When I did this he took only ten minutes to nod off, and I even began to enjoy our bedtime cuddle.

The amount and type of help that infants and young children need at sleep time varies from child to child. Some babies might be able to go to sleep by themselves at three months while their siblings need cuddling well into the second year. Sometimes babies will settle more easily at sleep time if their awake-time experiences help them feel confident of their parents' availability. When moms and dads predictably offer comfort when needed and encourage babies to enjoy their emerging independence, they can go to sleep knowing they are safe. Understanding that your baby needs *you* at sleep time (and at other times too!) is the first step toward responsive and sensitive parenting.

Touch and Emotional Health

Touching, holding, and rocking are great for your baby, both psychologically and physically. One research study found that babies who were held regularly by their mothers in a cloth sling were more than twice as likely to be securely attached to their mothers as babies who weren't.[4] Loving touch also enables children to feel close to their parents, fostering the development of an intimate relationship.[5]

Holding babies close and caressing them can lower the stress hormones circulating in their blood and help them cope 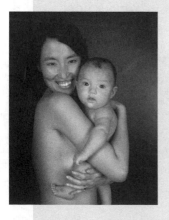 with upsetting or distressing events.[6] One study found that babies who were carried frequently by their parents cried and fussed about half as much as babies who weren't—including in the evening when many infants are very fussy.[7] Loving physical contact increases blood flow, improves breathing, digestion, and absorption of food, and helps the heart rate and rhythm develop optimally.[8] Touch can even release growth hormones that stimulate babies' body and brain growth![9]

Communication: Pay Attention to What Your Baby Is Trying to Tell You

Although they can't speak, babies and young children do use language to express their feelings, intentions, and needs—their behavior. One of the greatest gifts parents can give their babies is to pay attention to how they are behaving and *think* about what that behavior means.[10] Trying to figure out what babies are attempting to communicate helps them feel understood and lets them know they are important to you. And as you become more adept at decoding their behavior, you will be able to respond to their needs more efficiently. The following mother describes how recognizing what her son was trying to say helped her fulfill his needs at sleep time:

> After having two babies who were cuddled to sleep, I figured I had this mothering thing under control. Then along came number three. Jake was a very easygoing baby, but one day when he was only a few weeks old, I tried to cuddle him after his feed and waited for him to fall asleep. He wouldn't settle and kept arching his back to pull away from me. I changed positions, held him tighter, and rocked harder. This went on for a little while until in frustration, I put him down in his bed to give myself a break. He went straight to sleep!
>
> From that day forward, the best way to get him to sleep was to put him to bed. Through teething, sickness, and a few unsettled nights, he sometimes needed a little drink or a pat on the back. He was, and still is, a very cuddly child during the day, but if I picked him up to rock him to sleep he would always arch his back. It was his way of saying "Thanks, Mom, but I need my space now." Jake is now almost two and still likes his own space to sleep in. I've found that each child is an individual and needs to be nurtured and loved differently.

By thinking about what each of her children were telling her, this mother was able to meet each child's unique needs. The following questions will help you think about your own baby's sleep-time language:

- How does my baby tell me when he is tired?

- Have his tired signs changed over time?

- When I notice he's tired, how long do I wait before helping him to sleep? Does the length of this wait affect how easily he goes to sleep?

- How do I help him go to sleep? Which sleep techniques or bedtime routines have been the most successful? Which have been the least successful?

- How does my baby respond at these times? What is he trying to tell me with his responses?

It's Okay to Take Charge

Being a parent is like being in a continuous dance with your baby, except that the person who leads varies depending on the circumstances. Most often responsive parents follow their babies' lead, watching them closely to see what they need and responding warmly.[11] For instance, you might know that your baby is getting tired when her attention span shortens and she becomes easily frustrated, so you follow her lead and begin settling her down to sleep. At other times, though, parents need to take charge.[12] Fifteen-month-old Anna, for example, might think it's time to play with her blocks, but her parents know she's been hyperexcited for the past fifteen minutes—a sign it's definitely time for bed! They need to take the lead by gently coaxing her away from the blocks or, if that fails, picking her up and carrying her into the bedroom. Anna may howl and cry, but her parents know that by calming her with kind words and cuddles, she'll eventually finish protesting and settle down to sleep.

Some parents find it difficult to take charge, because they're afraid that setting limits will make their little ones resent them, or they're simply not sure what limits to set. Other parents desperately want their babies to need them, so they feel anxious at the thought of separating from them, even just to go to sleep. We suspect that for these parents, the prospect of sleep training may be liberating or appealing because it gives them a sense of certainty and much-needed permission to take charge at sleep time. But there are lots of ways to have rules while still meeting babies' needs for comfort and security. No book can tell you exactly how to achieve this: knowing when to lead and when to follow involves watching babies closely and seeing if they can manage the limits you're setting.

Your Actions: Realize How Your Behavior Affects Your Child

As a parent, you need to consciously and actively consider how your thoughts, feelings, and actions have an impact on your children. Imagine, for instance, a dad who comes home from work each night eager to play with his five-month-old daughter. He might engage in some of the "dad play" that babies love: scoop her up in his arms, tumble her around, and blow raspberries on her roly-poly legs. For some reason, however, each night after playing for a while, his baby starts to cry inconsolably for the next hour. Not surprisingly, Dad begins to feel like a failure and becomes frustrated by how long it takes his daughter to fall asleep.

If this father thought clearly about the situation, he might realize what is happening: He is preoccupied by the day's events and doesn't notice that his daughter is showing her tired signs. He might then recognize that he is playing with her according to his tempo, not hers. In this case, it would be best if Dad tried to unwind and put the day behind him before his arrival at home. He could help his daughter settle down, too, by giving her a massage and singing her lullabies. Playtime could be saved for morning. If this dad doesn't think about how his actions affect his daughter, he will continue to be bewildered by her behavior. He might begin to see her as a difficult or naughty baby, or hand over all the evening parenting to his partner, saying, "You do it—you're better at it than I am."

What you're thinking and how you're feeling both affect how you interact with your baby. This, in turn, influences how your child interacts with you—day *and* night. The more aware you become of your own mental states, emotions, and intentions, the better able you will be to consider the effect they have on your baby.

Empathy: Truly Understand Your Baby's Feelings

Empathy is the ability to sincerely understand what other people are feeling and experiencing. You can develop empathy for your baby by paying careful attention to his behavior and thinking about which needs and feelings he is attempting to communicate. When you have empathy for your child, you are more likely to respond to his crying: you can feel that he is sad, upset, or angry.[13] Empathic parents understand that when their child is frightened, he needs comfort and protection even if there is no apparent threat or danger.[14]

Showing empathy to your children is like wrapping them in soft warm blankets when they are shivering with cold; it helps them tolerate and recover from painful feelings.[15] As we saw in chapter 3, doing this repeatedly establishes the structures in babies' brains that allow them to calm themselves and regulate their feelings. Not only does empathy feel good for babies, it's also crucial to their emotional development.[16] It builds and strengthens the parts of their brains that enable them to really "get" what others are feeling. This type of emotional intelligence makes people better friends, more cooperative students and workers, and generally easier to get along with. Parents' thoughts about their babies sow the seeds of empathy in them. It's helpful to remember the following:

- Your baby really feels the emotions he shows, so if he sounds distressed, he is distressed, not merely tired.[17]

- Your baby's cries always signal genuine need and are always legitimate, regardless of whether the cause is physical or emotional.[18]

- Your baby has good intentions; she is not out to make your life difficult or to manipulate you.[19]

Recognizing genuine need can help parents tremendously when figuring out how to get their babies to sleep. One little girl would wake up the second she was put down for her daytime nap; although exasperated, her parents tried to understand her sleep-time needs to find a solution. Her mom explains:

> I felt incredibly frustrated. I didn't want to keep holding and rocking her while she slept, but I also didn't want her to wake up and be upset after being put down. Here is what worked for us after a lot of trial and error: a battery-operated baby swing. The movement lulled her to sleep. . . . For added benefit, we draped a used nursing bra over her chest so that she could have my smell.

This mother's empathy helped her understand her baby's needs at nap time—her daughter needed both movement and to feel that her mother was nearby. A creative sleep solution was the result.

Having empathy doesn't mean trying to *stop* your child's difficult feelings or crying: That can be like trying to stop a train hurtling down the tracks. It's more like sitting in the train cabin with your child until the end of the journey, so he doesn't feel so alone during the scary ride. In practice, this means providing comfort and reassurance that's right for your baby's level of distress.[20] For example, if you put your baby in his crib to sleep and he fusses a little bit, you might just pat his back and hum to him until he settles down. But if he is screaming and reaching out to you, he needs more comfort—probably to be picked up and cuddled.

Although it can be emotionally draining, consoling your babies when they feel sad is a great chance to help them feel secure and close to you. Think about the friends in your life: you may have good-time and casual friends, but those to whom you feel closest are those with whom you share your sadness and disappointments.

Repair Your Relationship with an Older Child

The six relationship skills described in this chapter apply to older children as well as babies. It is never too late to find new ways of helping your child feel accepted and secure even if your relationship had a rocky beginning. Psychologist Robert Karen says the following:

> To be understood instead of punished, to express anger and not be rejected, to complain and be taken seriously, to be frightened and not have one's fear trivialized, to be depressed or unhappy and feel taken care of, to express a self-doubt and feel listened to and not judged—such experiences may be for later childhood what sensitive responsiveness to the baby's cries and other distress signals are for infancy.[21]

There are some excellent books about meeting the emotional needs of toddlers and older children. If you're interested, check out "Suggested Reading" on pages 197 to 200.

Emotional Regulation: Manage Your Baby's Feelings

Most of us are pretty good at regulating our body temperature—if we're hot, we'll open a window or turn on the air conditioner; if we're cold, we'll put on a sweater or turn on the heat. However, when it comes to feelings, people's ability to regulate their emotional "temperature" varies enormously. Some people manage their feelings well: They are openly joyful, express their sadness, and freely share their disappointments with friends and family. For others, a healthy emotional balance is harder to achieve. Some are dominated by fiery, overpowering emotions and vacillate between excitement and despair, often immersing themselves in intense relationships and abruptly cutting off from those who are close to them. Others go through life being emotionally supercool—never getting too close to anyone and remaining unaware of their difficult feelings.

Babies are not born with the capacity to manage their feelings; emotional regulation is something children develop through their relationships with their parents.[22] Helping babies and children learn how to cope with their feelings is the emotional equivalent of making sure they have a roof over their heads and food in their tummies—it

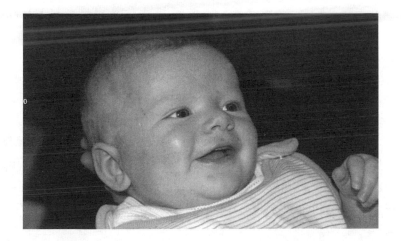

is that fundamental to their well-being. Strong emotional regulation skills are the hallmark of good mental health. Depression and anxiety disorders are a result of the brain's inability to regulate emotions.

Children who can manage their feelings well have a terrific head start. They have better concentration, make friends more easily, are good friends to others, can feel angry without becoming aggressive or violent, and are less prone to depression and anxiety. These children are also more likely to be cooperative and fun to have around.

But children only learn to understand and regulate their feelings if their parents respond well to their emotions most of the time. When parents consistently help their children identify their feelings and assist them to calm down after experiencing difficult emotions, over time children learn how to manage these feelings themselves.[23] They come to expect that someone will respond promptly when they feel sad or out of control, that they will be taken care of. This gives children the ability to contain anxiety and fall back on a sense of security; it instills confidence in them that things will soon be okay.[24] In chapter 3, we likened this to parents acting like training wheels— repeatedly helping children balance their emotions so eventually they learn how to balance themselves. Children who consistently receive this assistance are more likely to grow into secure, confident adults who can manage difficult feelings on their own and are less likely to become neurotic or anxious.[25] They will also be able to ask for help from others when their feelings become too overwhelming to handle by themselves.

Some parents may feel fear or even panic when their children are distressed or want comfort. They will do almost anything to downplay or distract their children from these feelings. Confronted with their babies howling in sadness, these parents shake toys in their faces rather than hold them close and stroke their heads. Downplaying or trying to distract children from their feelings does not help them settle down. More likely it sends the message that "feeling sad makes my parents uncomfortable. I'd better stop being open with them when I feel this way." In the future, these children can continue to hide their sadness from others who care about them, such as friends, teachers, and romantic partners. They may even unconsciously disconnect from these feelings, because being aware of them would be far too painful.

Children can process difficult feelings in a straightforward way when their parents accept their emotions, wait patiently while the feelings pass, and give comfort when needed. In the short term, children can truly return to a calm state; in the long term, they feel safe to express whatever they feel.

Talk to Your Baby about Feelings

A good way to help babies manage their feelings is to talk to them regularly about how they feel and why. Try to notice a whole range of feelings—positive and negative. For example, "You're grumpy because you just woke up and you want a big cuddle with Mommy to help you really feel awake." At first it might feel strange to do this, but many children—even young infants—calm down if you accurately describe what they're feeling, and over time they will become comfortable telling you what they feel and why.

Your Feelings: Look After Your Own Needs

In order to help your baby develop strong emotional regulation skills, you need to develop some emotional muscle yourself. This means being willing to experience and manage your feelings, including difficult ones. It's like teaching babies to swim: Just as you need to feel comfortable splashing around in water before you can help them learn to swim, you need to feel comfortable with all sorts of feelings before you can help babies be comfortable with theirs. According to psychologist Zeynep Biringen, "Some of the biggest problems in parent-child relationships arise when parents refuse to access their own emotions because they wish to avoid the pain of doing so."[26] For example, parents who dismiss their children's neediness or anger may fear, consciously or unconsciously, becoming emotionally vulnerable and being overwhelmed by these feelings.[27] If, however, parents can learn how to tolerate difficult feelings such as neediness and anger, they will be better able to help their children when they struggle with these same feelings.

When you were a child, if your parents made it clear that certain feelings were unwelcome visitors in your home, you may still feel uncomfortable dealing with these emotions. Do any of the following phrases sound familiar?

- "You're okay; cheer up."
- "It could be much worse."
- "There's nothing to be upset about."
- "What have you got to cry about?"
- "How can you be angry about that?"
- "You big scaredy-cat."
- "Don't be a crybaby."

These messages minimize or deny a child's feelings as well as the right to have these feelings. If this is how your parents responded to *your* sad or angry feelings, quite possibly you will find yourself saying the same kinds of things to your children. Psychologist Robert Karen explains:

> Many parents, because their own dependency needs were rebuffed as children, still live in unresolved pain over them. . . .

> Clinical evidence suggests that parents cannot tolerate seeing their unmet needs expressed by their children, and they cannot tolerate the anger and distress the child expresses when those needs go unmet again. . . . Perhaps because to be fully open to the baby's emotional needs is to become reacquainted with oneself as a baby, to re-experience the pain of being totally dependent and desperately in love and yet being shut out and feeling unwanted.[28]

Without conscious consideration of how your childhood experiences affect the way you think, feel, and behave, you are likely to treat your children just like your parents did you and may unintentionally pass on unhealthy relationship patterns.[29] Just becoming aware of your emotional makeup is a huge step toward change. No one is pretending that this is an easy journey; it's like being willing to travel to the South Pole even if you hate the cold. Pretty soon, though, and with practice, you can learn to tolerate these feelings— just as you would become acclimated to the cold. The greater the emotional terrain you can endure, the more help you will be to your baby. This is not to say that you need to spend years in therapy before you can be emotionally available to your baby, although counseling or therapy can certainly be helpful. It *does* mean that you need to be willing to acknowledge and confront any uneasy feelings that parenthood has stirred up for you.

According to psychiatrist Stanley Greenspan, "If your baby's anger, clinginess, or curiosity makes you feel uneasy, you can't ignore these feelings. Trying to do so merely drives them underground, where they tend to fester. The best way to defuse things is to honestly take stock of your own particular soft spots."[30] Apart from the long-term psychological advantages for your baby, being able to manage your feelings can have immediate benefits for you both: remember that the most important step in calming down your baby at sleep time is being able to calm yourself first.[31]

What if You Can't Bear to Hear Your Baby Cry?

Some health professionals tell parents there is something wrong with them if they can't tolerate the crying that comes with sleep training, sometimes even saying that they have a serious problem and need counseling. This is a heartless message and groundless too: parents find it difficult to listen to their babies cry because that is how their brains and biology are designed.

We offer one word of caution, though. If you feel highly anxious or even panicked whenever your baby cries, it would be worthwhile to think about the source of these feelings, as your baby will sense your panic. If you respond to your baby promptly but in a manner that is relaxed, rather than anxious and urgent, your baby will feel more confident that all is right with the world.

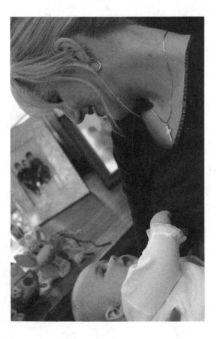

Secure Parents Raise Secure Children

Parents who were secure as children usually raise secure babies and children. And those who felt insecure but have resolved many of their childhood issues are also highly likely to be sensitive parents who raise secure children.[32] Whether you had a wonderful or a terrible childhood is not as significant to how secure your child feels as whether or not you have come to terms with what happened in your past.[33] Becoming conscious of how your childhood influences your parenting is neither quick nor easy. It is an ongoing process, but an important one. It allows us to enjoy richer and more rewarding relationships with our children. Your babies' relationship with you is the most important one they will ever have. Fostering your ability to relate to them emotionally is an investment in their future and in your lifetime connection with them.

Dealing with Unresolved Trauma— Crucial for Sensitive Parenting

Sadly, many parents have experienced some degree of trauma in their lives. They may have been sexually assaulted, lived in a war zone, been the victim of domestic violence, or lived with neglectful alcoholic parents. Memories of these events can be as excruciating as the events themselves, and it's understandable that some people cope by trying to ignore their past.

If these issues remain unresolved, however, they can have lives of their own, causing a person to dissociate under stress, for example, or lead a life of excessive rigidity or chaos.[34] This unresolved trauma can make it difficult for parents to be consistently emotionally available and sensitive to their children's cues. Babies and young children are exquisitely tuned in to their parents' emotions. They can be frightened by the expressions on their parents' faces that appear when traumatic experiences replay in their minds. One way children can express this fear is through somatic disturbances such as sleeping difficulties.

If you have unresolved trauma, we encourage you to do what you can to resolve this experience for yourself. Child psychiatrist Daniel J. Siegel and early childhood expert Mary Hartzell offer this advice in their book, *Parenting from the Inside Out*:

> *[Coming to terms with traumatic events] can be done in solitude, but it is often helpful to allow others to bear witness to our pain and our journey toward healing. Resolution depends upon the ability to be open and face what at times*

may seem like unbearable feelings. The good news is that healing is possible. Often the hardest step is acknowledging that there is some serious and frightening unresolved business. When we can take the deliberate steps to face the challenge of knowing the truth, we are ready to begin the path toward healing and growth and become more the parent we'd like to be.[35]

Not only will coming to terms with traumatic events improve your quality of life, it will also help you and your child enjoy a richer and closer relationship.

The following questions are designed to encourage you to think about your baby's feelings and how available you are to help with those feelings. (If you find that these questions raise any difficult emotions for you, we recommend you talk with your partner or a close friend, or seek the guidance of a skilled counselor.)

- How does my baby tell me when she is experiencing joy, sadness, fear, anger, or interest in the world?

- What thoughts and feelings do I have when my baby expresses her feelings?

- Are there any feelings I'm particularly uncomfortable with? Is this discomfort linked to my childhood in any way?

- How do I respond to my baby when she expresses emotions that I feel uncomfortable with?

- Is there any way I could better manage these difficult feelings for myself and better help my baby with these feelings?

Key Points

- Being an emotional resource for your child rests on six core relationship skills: recognizing how important you are to him, paying attention to what he is trying to tell you, realizing how your actions affect him, having empathy for his feelings, learning how to regulate his emotions, and looking after your own needs.

- Having empathy for your baby and sensitively helping her learn to manage her feelings have a profound, positive influence on her mental health.

- The way you were parented can affect how attuned you are to your children's emotional needs. It's very helpful to become aware of the impact your childhood has on your parenting style. Just realizing that your baby's behavior can stir up uncomfortable feelings in you is a big step toward becoming an emotionally responsive parent.

NOTES

1. Arietta Slade, "Keeping the Baby in Mind: A Critical Factor in Perinatal Mental Health," *Zero to Three* 10, no. 16 (June/July 2002): 15.

2. The first five skills described in this chapter have been adapted from the five "Relationship Capacities" as discussed in Glen Cooper, Kent Hoffman, Bert Powell, and Robert Marvin, "The Circle of Security Intervention: Differential Diagnosis and Differential Treatment," in *Enhancing Early Attachments: Theory, Research, Intervention, and Policy*, eds. Lisa J. Berlin, Yair Ziv, Lisa Amaya-Jackson, and Mark T. Greenberg (New York: Guilford Press, 2005), 127–151.

3. Cooper et al., "The Circle of Security Intervention," 127–151.

4. Elizabeth Anisfeld, Virginia Casper, Molly Nozyce, and Nicholas Cunningham, "Does Infant Carrying Promote Attachment? An Experimental Study

of the Effects of Increased Physical Contact on the Development of Attachment," *Child Development* 61, no. 5 (1990): 1617–1627.

5. Stanley Greenspan, with Nancy Breslau Lewis, *Building Healthy Minds: The Six Experiences that Create Intelligence and Emotional Growth in Babies and Young Children* (New York: Perseus, 1999).

6. Zeynep Biringen, *Raising a Secure Child: Creating an Emotional Connection Between You and Your Child* (New York: Berkley Publishing Group/ Penguin, 2004).

7. See note 4 above.

8. Richard M. Restak, *The Infant Mind* (New York: Doubleday, 1986).

9. Greenspan, with Lewis, *Building Healthy Minds*, 28.

10. Slade, "Keeping the Baby in Mind," 10–16.

11. Circle of Security: Early Intervention Program for Parents and Children, "Traveling Around the Circle of Security," www.circleofsecurity.net/ assests/forms_pdf/COS_travelingaroundCOS.pdf (accessed May 2009).

12. Ibid.

13. Debra M. Zeifman, "Predicting Adult Responses to Infant Distress: Adult Characteristics Associated with Perceptions, Emotional Reactions, and Timing of Intervention," *Infant Mental Health Journal* 24, no. 6 (2003): 597–612; and Vicky Flory, *Your Child's Emotional Needs: What They Are and How to Meet Them* (Sydney: Finch, 2005).

14. See note 3 above.

15. Colwyn Trevarthen, "Intrinsic Motives for Companionship in Understanding: Their Origin, Development, and Significance for Infant Mental Health," *Infant Mental Health Journal* 22, nos. 1–2 (2001): 95–131; and note 5 above.

16. Daniel N. Stern, *The Interpersonal World of the Infant: A View from Psychoanalysis and Developmental Psychology* (New York: Basic Books, 1985); and Zeifman, "Predicting Adult Responses to Infant Distress," 597–612.

17. Flory, *Your Child's Emotional Needs*.

18. Zeifman, "Predicting Adult Responses to Infant Distress," 597–612.

19. See note 17 above.

20. Margaret Hope, *For Crying Out Loud: Understanding and Helping Crying Babies* (Sydney: Sydney Children's Hospital, 1996).

21. Robert Karen, *Becoming Attached: First Relationships and How They Shape Our Capacity to Love* (New York: Oxford University Press, 1994), 243.

22. Circle of Security: Early Intervention Program for Parents and Children, "Treatment Assumptions," www.circleofsecurity.org/treatmentassumptions.html (accessed July 2008).

23. See note 3 above.

24. Carolyn Quadrio, "Controlled Crying," April 30, 2006.

25. Ibid.

26. Biringen, *Raising a Secure Child*, 43.

27. Richard A. Fabes, Stacie A. Leonard, Kristina Kupanoff, Carol Lynn Martin, et al., "Parental Coping with Children's Negative Emotions: Relations with Children's Emotional and Social Responding," *Child Development* 72, no. 3 (May 2001): 907–920

28. Karen, *Becoming Attached*, 243, 374.

29. See note 6 above; and Daniel J. Siegel and Mary Hartzell, *Parenting from the Inside Out: How a Deeper Self-Understanding Can Help You Raise Children Who Thrive* (New York: Jeremy P. Tarcher/Penguin, 2003).

30. Greenspan, with Lewis, *Building Healthy Minds*, 126.

31. See note 5 above.

32. Erik Hesse, "The Adult Attachment Interview: Historical and Current Perspectives," in *Handbook of Attachment: Theory, Research, and Clinical Applications*, eds. Jude Cassidy and Phillip R. Shaver (New York: Guilford Press, 1999), 395–433.

33. Biringen, *Raising a Secure Child*, 35; and Siegel and Hartzell, *Parenting from the Inside Out*.

34. Siegel and Hartzell, *Parenting from the Inside Out*.

35. Ibid., 139.

CHAPTER 8

Taking Care
of Yourself

Unless you receive emotional food, it is difficult
for you to cook up the same for your child.[1]
ZEYNEP BIRINGEN

We conclude this book with a chapter about parents and their needs. You deserve love and care just as much as your baby does. When you receive nurturing and practical help, you will enjoy being a parent more and will be better able to nurture your baby. And if your little one does have sleep problems, you definitely need a support team.

Being a parent is fantastic, but it can also be tiring and incredibly frustrating. When you were single and living it up, no one ever told you that you might end up so exhausted you couldn't remember what day it was, sitting on the couch at 1 P.M. in your pajamas feeling bored and lonely. Or that you would rush off to the office every morning with mashed baby food on one sleeve and a child clinging to the other. Parenting is never going to be a trouble-free job, but there are certainly ways to make it easier. In this chapter, we look at some of the things you can do to take care of yourself so you can really enjoy your child's early years.

Get Your Head *and* Heart in the Right Place

New moms and dads often feel very unsure and vulnerable. What are you supposed to do with this fragile little person who just joined your family? You want to be a good parent, so if professionals offer advice, you may well try what they recommend. One of the many reasons parents use sleep training is because they desperately need help and support—and sadly, too often they are advised to let their babies cry themselves to sleep.

Some parenting writers suggest that one of the ways to protect yourself from the whirlpool of bad advice is to trust your instincts, or follow your heart. This is good advice to a point, but if you're

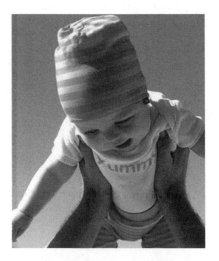

like many modern parents you might wonder exactly what your instincts are or just how you should follow your heart. Instinctive parenting is actually a whole lot easier if your head is in the right place first—that is, if you accept that parenthood has its share of both rewarding, enjoyable moments and challenging, frustrating ones. The following are a few things many parents wish they had been told *before* they had babies!

Relax and Enjoy Your Baby

Babies are fun. They're cute—when they smile and laugh, their whole bodies are consumed with happiness. Sometimes when you feel tired or depressed or you have fussy babies who are hard work, it is tough to remember to enjoy them. Yet even the most colicky baby has happy moments—catch her smiling and smile back. Look at how beautiful she is and tell her. Stare into her eyes and stroke her soft hair. Take a bath with her. Tickle and laugh with her. The following are some comments we heard from parents:

> I wish that we had spent more time just enjoying her and less time worrying about establishing a routine.

> All my children are now content and are good sleepers. I just wish I could have spent more quality time enjoying their neediness and not expecting so much from them as infants.

> You can enjoy life and be tired at the same time.

Accept That Every Baby Is Different

While we might all want easy babies—who are usually relaxed and happy, fall asleep quickly, sleep through the night from an early age, and spend most of the day laughing and cooing—the vast majority of babies are not like this. Most have difficult days, weeks, or even months. Some infants are just incredibly hard work most of the time.

We've mentioned Anni's second baby, Ben, a few times because he taught us a lot about the needs of sensitive babies. For instance, when Beth visited Anni's family, Ben cried at the mere sight of her—for him, a long-haired stranger was very scary. Part of the reason Anni found taking care of Ben so difficult was because she spent the first year thinking, "It shouldn't be this way," especially because she'd had a relatively easy time with her first baby, Zac. Other parents have shared this same experience:

> I was so focused on what she was "supposed" to be doing that instead of adapting to her needs, I tried to force her into doing what was not natural for her.

> Every child is different. . . . It is most important to work with the child you have and not with the child you wish you had!

> Don't stress about it: each baby will have [his or her] own
> unique rhythm and your life will be simpler and easier if you
> learn that rhythm and adapt to it.

Accepting the baby you have—not the baby you think you should have or the baby other people say you should have—will help you adjust to your child's needs and make everyone's life easier. Anni was much more relaxed with her third baby, Karl, because she had learned a crucial lesson: parents need to adapt to each baby they bring into the world.

Remember: This Too Shall Pass

When you're tired and adjusting to the whirlwind of changes—both welcome and unwelcome—that come with parenthood, it can feel like life will never be any different; that you will *always* be helping your child sleep and getting up through the night. But change is inevitable. Many people say this, but it's so true: Your child's babyhood will be over before you know it. Whatever sleep issues you and your baby are currently struggling with will pass with time and some creative thinking.

Sandy Jones, author of *Crying Baby, Sleepless Nights*, had a daughter who did not sleep for periods longer than three hours during the first two years of her life. She says, "In the early days of childrearing, it would have been a great relief to know that my baby's sleep problem would resolve itself in due time, that I would remember the nursing years with great tenderness, and that my daughter would turn out to be a bright, responsible, and sociable adult."[2] Babies' bedtime neediness will not go on forever—taking a loving and responsive approach in these early years is something you will never regret.

Is Your Baby's Sleep Really the Issue?

Parents can become obsessed with their babies' sleep, thinking that if only they slept better everything would be okay. Sometimes babies' sleep may appear to be the problem, but on deeper examination other issues are actually at the heart of parents' stress. Consider this mother's story:

> My first two daughters were quite wakeful as babies, and I was very tired for what felt like a very long time! While this was difficult to cope with, with the benefit of hindsight, I can see that there were other things happening in my life that greatly exacerbated the problem. The first was my partner's undiagnosed postnatal [postpartum] depression, which left me feeling terribly emotionally unsupported. This isolation was compounded by having very few friends in my neighborhood, which meant that I spent many long days at home without speaking to another adult. While much has changed for the better in our life, I wish that we had been able to address my partner's depression earlier, and that I had been able to find a community of other mothers to connect with sooner. I am certain this would have made my tiredness 100 percent easier to deal with.

It's worth taking time to carefully consider how your circumstances may have an impact on how you're coping with parenthood. Looking at the whole picture may help you see your situation in a new light.

Rest Assured That Your Efforts Will Pay Off

Knowing how important you are to your child can feel like a burden at times. Choosing to respond to your baby's cries means that, in the short term, you may be more tired than parents who use sleep training or turn off the baby monitor at night. It's easy to wonder whether all of your efforts are worth it as you wake, bleary-eyed, already thinking about whether you can catch a nap that day.

Yet this knowledge is also a blessing. By responding to your baby when he needs you, you are teaching him to expect that you will be there for him no matter what. Over time this feeling enables him to feel lovable, secure, and safe. Through making yourself available to your child, you are helping him learn to think, "I'm a good person. I'm worth helping. I can get the help I need." Day by day (and night by night), you are building a solid foundation for your babies' mental and emotional health, and also strengthening their relationship with you.

In a way, responding to your children's cries is also a selfish act in the long term. The stronger the trust between you and your child, the easier it will be to navigate and overcome difficult periods in your relationship. As one mother commented, "My children have been relatively easy as they have grown older, and I firmly believe it is because of the way I parented them as babies."

Brainstorm Ways to Connect with Your Baby

The following questions will help you generate some ideas of how to get your head and heart in the right place:

- What are some moments with my child that I enjoy? (This week, jot down all the little things you adore about your baby; for example, "When I feed him, I notice how sweet and soft his little fingers are.")

- Are there any ways I could spend more time enjoying my beautiful baby?

- What activities and games does my baby really enjoy? Do I fully engage with her and share in her joy and delight when we play these games? Can we play these games together more often?

- Are there any new games or activities that I could try with my baby? (For example, singing along or dancing to a CD of children's songs together.)

- How can I reevaluate my current situation to help myself feel more relaxed? Do I remind myself often that all of the hard work I'm doing now will help my child feel closer and more connected to me in the future?

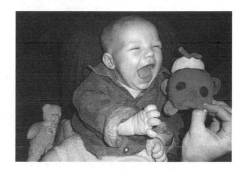

- Do I enjoy the fun, pleasurable moments I experience with my baby? Am I grateful for the precious gift of parenthood?

Seek Support and Advice from Good Sources

Once you put your head and heart in the right place, you are in a position to receive support and advice. When it comes to support, some parents are lucky enough to have extended family close by to help raise their children. Many of us are not so fortunate. Erika said this about living in Australia after spending several years in Ethiopia:

> Sometimes I feel quite isolated and lonely. I find in Western society that people can be too busy with their own lives. How many friends do you know whose parents offer little help with the grandchildren? In Ethiopia, the family structure is very strong. There is an established system in which family members assist each other. As a mother you would without question receive help from the female members of your family. If you had other children, they too would be expected to help both with the baby and around the house.

For all our technological sophistication and labor-saving devices, nothing is the same as having actual people around to help with our children and keep us company. In the Western world, however, it looks like the nuclear family is here to stay, so parents need to be imaginative to get the support they need.

Establish a Support System

When children are young, parents often struggle on a daily basis with all the demands placed on them. All families need support: extra arms to hold the baby, extra hands to cook the meals and do the housework, and extra time to rest and recover. We also need supportive connections with others: people to say hello to and chat with and people who care for us. Ideally we'd all have lots of family and friends close by and have good relationships in our local or spiritual community. Sadly, many of us have only a few of these supports—and some parents can raise their babies virtually alone. Also, parents don't always make the best use of the support available: they think that they should manage things by themselves or they aren't sure exactly what kind of support to seek or how to go about finding it.

It's helpful to look at areas of your life where you'd like some support and then take steps to put this support in place. Take a moment to think about the times when you are most stressed and exhausted—perhaps when you arrive home from work or on the weekends when you're juggling errands and activities. Next, try to figure out what kinds of support could help you manage in these situations: Could someone watch your baby while you take a nap in the afternoon? Could someone look after your older children when your baby requires your full attention? Could someone help out with the housework or preparing meals? Having a support team in place can make life so much easier!

Communicate with Your Partner and Support Each Other

When a baby joins a household, it means work—and lots of it. Our (very scientific) estimation is that each baby brings about 1000 percent increase in physical work (feeding, washing, changing, playing, cleaning up the various messes that baby gleefully makes on an hourly basis, and so on) and about the same increase in emotional work (soothing, comforting, settling to sleep, and so on). When coupled with a significant decrease in income (either from child care costs or the loss of the stay-at-home parent's income), this usually means much less "me time" and "us time."

There is pressure to earn income, pressure to get to work, and pressure to find a child care arrangement that is a good fit for your family. And staying at home with baby can easily leave the stay-at-home parent feeling isolated and lonely. Conflict and resentment can arise as partners struggle to understand each other's perspective and new needs. In general though, conflicts are likely to be short-lived if:

- each parent shares in the increased physical workload (even if one parent is also in full-time paid employment);

- each parent tries hard to understand and fulfill the needs of the other;

- both parents do their best to communicate without blame when conflicts arise;

- both parents see taking care of baby as an important and often very difficult job;

You will get along much better if you and your partner do your best to empathize with each other's challenges and take time to appreciate one another: remember, you love this person!

If You Think You or Your Partner May Be Depressed

New motherhood is a risky time for depression: about 20 percent of women suffer from postpartum depression, and dads can get postpartum depression too. Signs of depression include: taking no pleasure in your life or your baby; feeling sad and despondent day after day; feeling constantly angry and frustrated; feeling hopeless and helpless; thinking that you are a failure; thinking about harming yourself or your baby; and struggling to get out of bed each morning. Postpartum depression is also very hard on babies because they rely on their parents to share their happy feelings. If one or both parents cannot do this, a baby's emotional development can be affected.

Luckily, many excellent services are available to help people with postpartum depression. Ask your doctor for a referral to a postpartum depression support service (if there's one in your area). If your doctor can't help, see another one. The phone book and Internet should also have a list of resources in your area. If you're worried that a friend or partner is depressed, share your concerns with them and encourage them to seek help.

Ask for Help

Asking for help is the first step in getting the support you need. If you have a partner, you may want to start there. You could begin by making time for each other to refuel or relax (with exercise, enjoyable activities, and so on) or by asking for help to cook meals for the week or to spend time with you reorganizing your finances. Then look at joining local organizations, such as a mothers' group, or free services, such as a home visiting service. (Many excellent programs are available, especially to families with lower levels of income—see page 200 for some specific suggestions.) After this, provided you have the money, consider hiring help or signing up for activities; this is easy too—look up the cleaner's number or the yoga center and go for it. Some services such as gyms may have child care services on-site.

Finally, work with family and friends on the other areas you need support. Asking for unpaid help can feel a bit awkward because it is not something most of us are used to doing. It is best to state explicitly what you need and why and give the person a clear avenue to say no. For example, you could call your mother and say, "Hi, Mom. You know how Joshua is teething at the moment and needs a lot of cuddles?

Well it's really wearing me out, and the house is a mess. I was wondering if you could spare half a day for the next few weeks to come and give me a hand? It would really help, Mom, but I'll understand if you are too busy." Lots of people (even those you don't necessarily know so well) are happy to help—they just need to be given the opportunity to do so. For instance, asking for your neighbor's help might go like this: "Hi there. My baby is sick today and I can't get out of the house— I was wondering if you could pick me up a couple of things from the store?"

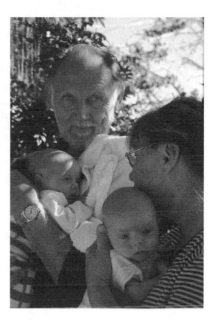

The following are some ways in which parents have sought the support they needed from their families, friends, and communities:

- Four families organized a cooking team: each family cooked one large meal on the weekends, split the meal into four, and shared it with the other three families.

- A mother paid a fifteen-year-old girl to come in each afternoon to cook dinner.

- One couple asked the mother's parents for some money so that she could take a year off work to look after the baby.

- A group of parents organized a house-helping roster: each week, one person helped out at someone else's house for a couple of hours.

- When the child of a single mom was diagnosed with a serious illness, neighbors cooked for the family and cared for the garden for two months.

- Parents have started playgroups by advertising in the local paper (you can specify what kinds of parents you want to hang out with; for example, younger moms, single dads, and so on).

- Parents with children of similar ages have created informal support groups by arranging for their children to play together regularly.

Remember that you're not being selfish by asking for help and support—making your life a little easier will mean that you're more able to fulfill your babies' needs. Take this opportunity to ask for the help you need. Make the call or send the email, and see what happens.

Come to Terms with Your Baby's Birth

The transition to motherhood can be very rocky—or even traumatic. Some women feel highly distressed following a birth over which they felt they had no control, and they may experience flashbacks, nightmares, and panic attacks.[3] Birth trauma can affect fathers too. These parents' ordeal is often compounded by well-meaning friends and family who say, "Just be happy that you have a healthy baby." This response can make parents feel like their loved ones are minimizing or discounting their painful experience.

If you feel upset about the birth of your baby, you deserve to be able to talk about it with someone who will acknowledge and validate your experience. If you do not have a friend or family member who can help you in this way, seek the services of a warm and skilled counselor. Good information on birth trauma can also be found in books, such as Sheila Kitzinger's *Birth Crisis* (New York: Routledge, 2006), and on websites such as www.birthtraumaassociation.org.uk and www.sheilakitzinger .com/BirthCrisis.htm.

Become Part of a Community

Finally, making the effort to become part of a community can help you feel more connected to others and expand your support team. When you were fully focused on work, a lot of your social contact may have come from your colleagues, so you may feel especially isolated without these interactions. Whether you are still in paid work or at home full-time, joining local activities allows you to form new connections.

There are lots of fantastic, enriching groups for parents of young children, such as playgroups and mothers' groups (and fathers' groups). Organizations or programs that are designed to educate parents on a specific topic, such as breast-feeding, young motherhood, fostering or adopting, developmental disability, or multiple births, offer many chances to connect with other parents (including those who might have gone through what you're going through) and to discuss general parenting topics. They can also provide access to libraries of useful parenting resources. Try going online to research appropriate groups and organizations in your area. Many cities also have free local parenting newspapers with good information about available resources and programs.

If you prefer to do something less focused on children, there are lots of opportunities as well. For example, you can join a scrapbooking, reading, or gardening group. Libraries, local newspapers, community centers, town halls, and the Internet are all great sources that can help you find groups that might be of interest. And if you can't get someone to look after your baby, oftentimes you can bring him or her along.

Volunteering is also an excellent way to feel like a meaningful part of a community. With some research, you can probably find opportunities that match a passion of yours (for example, environmental conservation or animal welfare). Look online at websites such as www.volunteermatch.org, or check your local newspaper for community groups seeking volunteers.

Consider Your Child Care Options

Many parents are happy to return to paid employment soon after their baby is born, and are able to make satisfactory child care arrangements. Others have a very limited maternity leave and find the thought of returning to work stressful, either because they are not ready to leave their baby or they are not satisfied with the child care available.

If you are not yet ready to leave your baby, consider what options may be feasible for you. Are you able to negotiate a longer period of unpaid leave once your maternity leave ends? Are part-time or job-share opportunities available? Could you work from home? Do you or your partner have vacation or other leave available? Could you work longer but fewer shifts? Do you have the opportunity to leave your job and return to the paid workforce at a later date?

If finding adequate child care is the issue, take time to make the best arrangements you possibly can. Could a family member look after your baby until you feel she is old enough for day care? Could you share the cost of a babysitter with one or two other families?

If you feel that day care is best for your child, make sure you are happy with the available care. Visit several child care centers, and take time to observe how staff members interact with the children. Are they warm, loving, and responsive? Do the children appear happy and well cared for? Consider how many caregivers exist per child—the lower the caregiver/child ratio, the more attention your child is likely to receive. Find out about the training and education of the caregivers. Is there low staff turnover and the opportunity for your child to bond with one or two consistent caregivers? Are staff members happy to give your child expressed breast milk if you're continuing to breast-feed? Do they respond kindly and sensitively to your questions and concerns?

Taking the time to make the best care arrangements for your child and family will help minimize everyone's stress level.

Find Helpful and Valid Advice

Unwanted advice is an occupational hazard when you're a parent. You may feel you're going along swimmingly until your aunt says "Breast-feeding him *again*, dear?" and you deflate like a balloon. Or you may want advice about a problem you're having but don't like the advice you receive.

Luckily, resources are available to you. Many wonderful health professionals are able to provide parents with support while at the same time keep babies' emotional needs in mind. If you receive advice that you feel does not respect your baby's emotional needs, we encourage you to search elsewhere. "Suggested Reading" (pages 197–200) lists books that offer helpful and sound advice, so these can be a good place to start. There are also many websites where parents can communicate and give each other advice and support. These cater to every sort of parent: single moms, single dads, foster parents, adoptive parents—whoever you are, there will be other parents like you chatting away in forums. The advice is variable, so be wary. And of course, remember that what works for other people's babies may not work for yours. But it is nice to have someone from the same city or the other side of the world say, "Hang in there; you're doing a good job!"

Brainstorm Ways to Reduce Stress

The following questions are designed to help you think about what causes stress in your life and what kind of support could alleviate the pressure:

- In which areas of my life could I really benefit from some support? What types of support would make a substantial difference to me? (Try to be specific.)
- Who could provide me with this support? Who could possibly help out in some way, even if it were only once a month? Would it be helpful to plan how I will make this request?

- How could my partner and I work together to support each other and fulfill each other's needs? Is there any way we could take time just for ourselves to nurture each other? (Write down something you could do each week for just the two of you.)

- How do I feel most of the time? (If you feel depressed, or upset about your birth experience, write down a list of people you could turn to for help. If you think counseling might be a good idea, ask your pediatrician, primary care physician, family nurse practitioner, or friends to recommend a psychologist or counselor.)

- Do I enjoy satisfying social connections with others? If not, what actions could I take to feel more connected to people in my community? When could I take these actions?

- Are there any services I could approach or organizations I could join? How would I go about doing this? What do I hope to gain or learn from them?

- Am I facing any problems or situations that I'm unable to resolve or handle on my own? Where might I find advice to help me cope?

- If I'm not comfortable with advice I've received, what new avenues could I pursue to find alternative advice?

Give the Gift of Listening

If you're the partner or friend of a tired parent, the simple act of listening can be enough to help him or her feel better. This sounds easy enough, but many people think that being a good listener means trying to solve someone's problems, when it really involves trying to understand someone's experience. The following are a few hints to keep in mind during your conversations with a tired parent:

- Listen for at least fifteen minutes before offering a solution.

- Don't rush to fill in any silences in the conversation. If you wait a few seconds, the person you're listening to will likely continue his or her story.

- Ask questions like: How does that affect you? What's that like for you? How do you feel when that happens? How can I support you? Then stop and really listen to the answers.

Skilled listening can act like a soothing balm to an agitated nervous system. It helps people express their feelings and think more clearly about their situation—they might even come up with creative solutions they hadn't thought of before.

Manage Temporary Tiredness

Many times in our lives, we feel almost constantly tired: when we're studying intensively, partying hard, working long days to meet an urgent deadline, ill, dealing with a crisis, or when we simply haven't had a vacation for far too long. And of course, when we have a baby. Many parents continue to feel tired even after their children start sleeping through the night; looking after active toddlers and children is demanding work, especially when combined with paid employment and running a household.

Being a parent is a time in your life when taking care of yourself—and allowing yourself to be taken care of—is important. This is true whether you are staying at home with your children or in full-time paid employment. Beth found that it was helpful to give herself permission to take it easy on those days when she felt really exhausted. Forgetting the housework, postponing nonurgent phone calls, planning an easy dinner—whatever she could do to slow down and enjoy her children—helped. On the days she went to work, she would take time to relax by reading a good book on the bus. Anni found that ordering groceries online meant she didn't have to spend energy going shopping, and that getting a half-hour nap in the afternoon allowed her to cope much better in the evening. The following are other ways in which parents have managed their tiredness:

> Catnap when you can; sleep when your baby sleeps during the day.

> Twice a week I meet a friend at 6 A.M. for a 45-minute walk. This makes such a difference as to how I feel during the day.

> See if you can change your work times—either cutting back on your hours or starting earlier or finishing later, so you can have a little time for yourself.

> My husband would get up and take over from 5 A.M., then I would sleep (unless baby needed a feed) until 7:30 A.M.

> I make sure to eat fresh, healthy food, as this gives me a lot of energy and helps me feel good about myself.

> Leave the baby with a trusted adult for a few hours and switch off from the twenty-four-hour on-call parenting gig.

Some parents find it difficult to sleep when their baby sleeps, but still take the opportunity to rest, meditate, or listen to relaxation tapes. Others find that preparing dinner in the morning makes the end of the day, when everybody is the most tired, run more smoothly.

Many parents think that they should be able to cope on their own with the demands of parenthood, running a household, and generating income. Yet all parents need and deserve support to do this amazing—but seriously challenging—job. Being a parent is not easy; at times it's tiring, frustrating, and boring. Yet in life, many of our most worthwhile achievements have been the hardest. We feel proud when we meet the rigors of a new job, persist through a difficult course of study, or survive a rough patch with a partner. Challenges in life—such as managing the stresses of parenting—often teach us that we are more capable than we ever knew. Sometimes we can feel so overwhelmed that we forget to step back and think about some simple actions that could recharge and refuel us. The following questions are designed to help you consider what you can do to reduce your tiredness:

- How often do I eat fresh, healthy food? (Write down some ways that you could incorporate healthier food into your diet.)

- How often do I exercise? (Write down a range of twenty-minute physical activities you could do every day and when you could start doing them.)

- How often do I take a moment to relax and escape from the demands of my day? (Write down a list of calming activities you could do every day and when you could start doing them.)

- What else could I do to feel better rested, and when could I start doing these things?

Key Points

- All parents need—and deserve—lots of support.

- Keep the following advice in mind: relax and enjoy your baby; accept that every baby is different; remember that things will get better; and rest assured that your efforts will pay off both in terms of your child's development and his relationship with you.

- If you think the advice you receive is insensitive to your baby's needs, look elsewhere. There is a lot of good advice available from professionals, books, and websites.

- Think creatively about how to get the support you need to cope with temporary tiredness.

NOTES

1. Zeynep Biringen, *Raising a Secure Child: Creating an Emotional Connection Between You and Your Child* (New York: Berkley Publishing Group/Penguin, 2004), 147.

2. Sandy Jones, *Crying Baby, Sleepless Nights: Why Your Baby Is Crying and What You Can Do About It*, Revised (Boston: Harvard Common Press, 1992), xii.

3. Sheila Kitzinger, *Birth Crisis* (New York: Routledge, 2006).

Afterword

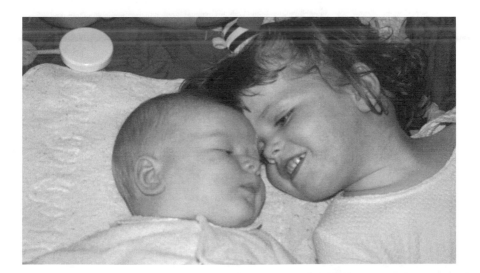

If I know what love is, it is because of you.[1]
HERMANN HESSE

The importance of early emotional experiences in the development of children's personalities and resilience is now irrefutable. Children whose cries are responded to promptly and sensitively are happier and more secure than those whose cries are ignored. In this book, we explore just how much babies need their parents—they are designed to grow and mature under the continual loving guidance of their mothers and fathers. Little children are ill equipped to cope with scary and difficult feelings of fear, anxiety, and distress about being separated from Mom or Dad. Without help to deal with these emotions, babies are left struggling.

When babies have assistance to manage these feelings, they learn to trust and expect that their parents will be there for them whenever needed. Sleep training has the opposite effect on children; it denies them the type of parenting that they need to feel secure and regulate their emotions. It is never a loving act.

We now have a new understanding of just how crucial parents' love is to neurological and emotional development: Far from being a soft and nebulous concept, "love" is a vital instigator in making a baby's brain build connections and grow. Gentle, loving parenting enables emotional resilience and a strong stress response system so that our children, once grown, can deal robustly with life's challenges.

As in so many areas of life, modifying babies' sleep patterns is not likely to come quickly or easily, and parents need support to patiently work toward change while trying to enjoy their children. We are pleased that a growing number of organizations see the need for this type of support and that it is gradually becoming more available to families.

We will leave you with a recommendation from Mary Ainsworth, the most influential researcher in the history of developmental psychology:

> My advice to parents is not to miss an opportunity to show affection to their babies.[2]

Remember this advice at sleep time too.

NOTES

1. Hermann Hesse, *Narcissus and Goldmund* (New York: Picador, 2003).

2. Mary Ainsworth, quoted at the Circle of Security Workshop (Parramatta, Australia, March 16–17, 2006), presented by Glen Cooper and organized by the New South Wales Institute of Psychiatry.

Suggested Reading

The books prefaced by an asterisk (*) may not be readily available in the United States, which means that you might have to devote some extra time and energy to finding them. We recommend checking Amazon.com and Amazon.co.uk, or ordering directly from the author's or publisher's website. Although these titles are a bit harder to track down, we definitely think that they're worth the added effort and postage.

1: Why Babies Wake through the Night

Kellymom, "Parenting: Nighttime & Sleep," www.kellymom.com/parenting/sleep/index.html.

La Leche League International, www.llli.org.

William Sears, "8 Infant Sleep Facts Every Parent Should Know," www.askdrsears.com/html/7/t070200.asp.

William Sears, *Nighttime Parenting: How to Get Your Baby and Child to Sleep*, Revised (New York: Plume/Penguin, 1999).

2: Why Babies Need Their Parents at Sleep Time

Robert Karen, *Becoming Attached: First Relationships and How They Shape Our Capacity to Love* (New York: Oxford University Press, 1998).

3: Building Your Baby's Brain Day and Night

Sue Gerhardt, *Why Love Matters: How Affection Shapes a Baby's Brain* (New York: Brunner-Routledge, 2004).

Daniel J. Siegel and Mary Hartzell, *Parenting from the Inside Out: How a Deeper Self-Understanding Can Help You Raise Children Who Thrive* (New York: Jeremy P. Tarcher/Penguin, 2003).

Zero to Three, www.zerotothree.org.

4: Why Sleep Training Is Bad Advice

*Sheila Kitzinger, *Understanding Your Crying Baby: Why Babies Cry, How Parents Feel, What You Can Do About It* (London: Carroll & Brown, 2005).

Margot Sunderland, *The Science of Parenting: How Today's Brain Research Can Help You Raise Happy, Emotionally Balanced Children* (New York: Dorling Kindersley/Penguin, 2006).

5: Gentle Approaches to Help Your Baby Sleep

*Pinky McKay, *Sleeping Like a Baby: Simple Sleep Solutions for Infants and Toddlers* (Melbourne, Australia: Penguin, 2006).

James J. McKenna, *Sleeping with Your Baby: A Parent's Guide to Cosleeping* (Washington, D.C.: Platypus Media, 2007).

William Sears, Robert Sears, James Sears, and Martha Sears, *The Baby Sleep Book: The Complete Guide to a Good Night's Rest for the Whole Family* (New York: Little, Brown and Company/Hachette, 2005).

Ask Dr. Sears, www.askdrsears.com.

6: Common Sleep Problems— and How to Cope with Them

Harvey Karp, *The Happiest Baby on the Block: The New Way to Calm Crying and Help Your Newborn Baby Sleep Longer* (New York: Bantam Dell/Random House, 2003).

*Pinky McKay, *100 Ways to Calm the Crying* (South Melbourne, Australia: Lothian Books, 2002).

Pinky McKay, official website, www.pinky-mychild.com.

Elizabeth Pantley, *The No-Cry Sleep Solution: Gentle Ways to Help Your Baby Sleep Through the Night* (New York: McGraw-Hill, 2002).

Elizabeth Pantley, *The No-Cry Sleep Solution for Toddlers and Pre-schoolers: Gentle Ways to Stop Bedtime Battles and Improve Your Child's Sleep* (New York: McGraw-Hill, 2005).

Elizabeth Pantley, official website, www.pantley.com/elizabeth.

7: Responsive Parenting— Six Gifts You Can Give Your Child

*Zeynep Biringen, *Raising a Secure Child: Creating an Emotional Connection Between You and Your Child* (New York: Berkley Publishing Group/Penguin, 2004).

*Vicky Flory, *Your Child's Emotional Needs: What They Are and How to Meet Them* (Sydney: Finch, 2005).

Stanley Greenspan, with Nancy Breslau Lewis, *Building Healthy Minds: The Six Experiences that Create Intelligence and Emotional Growth in Babies and Young Children* (New York: Perseus, 2000).

*Pinky McKay, *Parenting by Heart: Unlock Your Intuition and Nurture with Confidence* (Port Melbourne, Australia: Lothian Books, 2001).

8: Taking Care of Yourself

Stephanie Dowrick, *Choosing Happiness: Life & Soul Essentials* (New York: Jeremy P. Tarcher/Penguin, 2005).

*Sheila Kitzinger, *The Year After Childbirth: Enjoying Your Body, Your Relationships, and Yourself in Your Baby's First Year* (New York: Charles Scribner's Sons, 1994).

Sarah Napthali, *Buddhism for Mothers: A Calm Approach to Caring for Yourself and Your Children* (Sydney: Allen & Unwin, 2003).

BabyCenter, "Mothers' Groups: How to Find One That Suits You," www.babycenter.com/0_mothers-groups-how-to-find-one-that-suits-you_11800.bc#articlesection2.

National Head Start Association, www.nhsa.org.

Nurse-Family Partnership, www.nursefamilypartnership.org.

Parents as Teachers, www.parentsasteachers.org.

Index

About the Authors

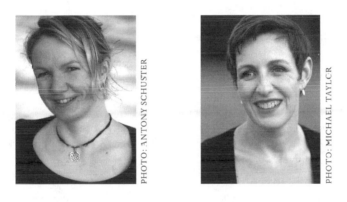

PHOTO: ANTONY SCHUSTER

PHOTO: MICHAEL TAYLOR

Anni Gethin, PhD, is a health social scientist with special interests in early childhood development and health equity. She runs a research and planning consultancy, lectures in public health and social science, and is the mother of three boys.

Beth Macgregor is a psychologist who trains health and welfare workers in infant mental health, child development, and child protection. She has worked as a child protection caseworker, specialist, and researcher, and is an active member of the Australian Association for Infant Mental Health. Her work as a specialist educator is devoted to creating happier children, families, and societies. Beth is the mother of two delightful little boys.

Both authors live in Sydney, Australia.